Scottish Medical Societies
1731–1939

Scottish Medical Societies
1731–1939
Their History and Records

JACQUELINE JENKINSON

EDINBURGH UNIVERSITY PRESS

Edinburgh University Press Ltd
22 George Square, Edinburgh

Typeset in Linotron Ehrhardt
by Koinonia Ltd, Bury, and
printed in Great Britain by
The University Press, Cambridge

A CIP record for this book is available from
British Library

ISBN 07486 0390 5

For My Mother and My Brothers and Sisters

Acknowledgements

I would like to take the opportunity to record my great debt to Anne Crowther and Marguerite Dupree for their guidance, help, and encouragement in the preparation of this book. My appreciation also goes to Brenda White whose brainchild this project was. Thanks also go to all the members of staff of the Glasgow Wellcome Unit for the History of Medicine, and the Modern History Department of Glasgow University, in particular, the late Geoffrey Finlayson.

The assistance of the archivists of the Grampian, Greater Glasgow, Lothian and Tayside Health Boards; of Aberdeen, Dundee, Edinburgh, Glasgow and Strathclyde Universities; and of the Royal College of Physicians, Edinburgh; are gratefully acknowledged, as is the assistance of the librarian of the Royal College of Physicians and Surgeons, Glasgow.

I appreciate the help of the librarians and staff of the following institutions: National Library of Scotland, Edinburgh; Wellcome Institute Library, London; Central Regional Council Archives, Stirling; North East Fife District Museums Service, Cupar; Victoria Infirmary, Glasgow; and the Royal Medical Society, Edinburgh.

I would also like to thank all the representatives of the many medical societies who assisted in this project, including: Alexander Adam; Allan A. Barclay; John Blair; Iain Boyle; John Calder; J. H. Drewer; Lesley Duncan; Donald Henry; James Innes; Isobel Kirkwood; William A. Liston; John McCracken; Charles McEwen; John McEwen; I. F. MacLaren; W. G. Middleton; Marion Rankin; Stefan Slater; Ian Syme; A. D. Toft; Ian Troup; and Arthur Wightman.

The research for this book was made possible by a grant from the Wellcome Trust.

The Carnegie Trust for the Universities of Scotland and the Scottish Society of the History of Medicine generously contributed to the cost of publication.

Contents

Part One

The History of Scottish Medical Societies
1731–1939

Introduction

Where two or more physicians or surgeons are employed in treating the same patient, or in making the same experiment, it is to be wished they would write the case or account of the experiment conjunctly, or at least that he who relates it would do it with all fairness and ingenuity, without discovering partiality for his own opinion, or disputing against the sentiments of others.[1]

(Introduction to Volume 1 of *Medical Essays and Observations* by a 'Society in Edinburgh', 1732)

Dr Mortimer (Turiff) brought before the meeting, the question 'Whether a medical man had a right to apply for a situation, which, at the time, was held by others, and where no vacancy existed, and whether he did not by so doing, commit a breach of professional etiquette.'[2]

(Extract from the minute book of the Garioch and Northern Medical Association, 1889)

Dr Walker Downie then exhibited a portion of a Brazil Nut which had become impacted in the right bronchus of a child, and after giving particulars of the case, described the method employed in its removal by trachiotomy.[3]

(Extract from the minute book of the Medico Chirurgical Society of Glasgow, 1892)

On Resections
We can do without stomach regards of intestine
and feeding without them is not work 'tis resting
A man may be a man with no legs underneath
and woman a woman sans eyes, tongue or teeth.[4]

(Final verse of an anonymous poem composed by a member of the Dundee Clinical Club on the occasion of the Club's 100th meeting, 1903)

As these quotations show, the activities of medical societies ranged from the educational through the professional to the convivial. This book aims, however, to do more than describe society activities. It is intended to serve two purposes: to be a general history of the 160[5] medical societies which existed between 1731 and 1939; and a guide to the individual societies including information about their formation, purposes, size, and the location of their surviving records. Both goals are important. First, relatively little has been written about the general role of medical societies in the development of the medical profession in Scotland, or in Great Britain as a whole.[6] The majority of existing studies[7] tend to focus on an individual society, and within that institution on its most famous members or important meetings. The emphasis in this work is on the wider context of the formation of individual societies; the variety of roles of the societies; and the relationship of the societies with the wider medical world.

The second part of this book lists each medical society in alphabetical order and provides a brief outline of the nature of the society : its size; frequency and content of its meetings; level of subscription for its members; whether it published transactions; the location of its records where extant; and a list of secondary publications and citations. The list includes both surviving and defunct societies.

Since the development of the medical profession in Scotland is reflected in the rise of medical societies, it is important to make clear at the outset of this book what is meant by the term 'profession', both in a general sense, and as it may be related to the historical development of medical practice in this period. There are various sociological interpretations of what defines a profession, and some of these provide a valuable insight into the subject. One of the earliest and most influential studies of the professions, written by Carr-Saunders and Wilson in 1930, describes the importance of association between fellow-practitioners in the development of professional identity. 'A profession can only be said to exist when there are bonds between the practitioners, and these bonds can take but one shape – that of formal association'[8]. 'Formal association' could also be used as a means of excluding 'irregular' – i.e. unqualified – practitioners from group recognition. Just as important as self-recognition within a professional body is public perception of the profession as a common body. 'The attention of the public is called to the existence of a profession through its professional association, and public recognition can hardly be accorded to a group which has not discovered itself.'[9]

The emphasis placed by Carr-Saunders and Wilson on professional association applies in the case of the profession of medicine in Scotland, albeit at an earlier date than they suggest for the emergence of professional associations nationally.

> The earliest professional associations of the modern type, dating from the late eighteenth and early nineteenth centuries, and often founded as dining clubs, were akin to the social, philanthropic, or learned society or workmen's club; and they assumed the form of a voluntary unincorporated association which all clubs adopted at that period...[10]

This quotation, by implication, places medical societies firmly in the vanguard of voluntary group activity which characterised social and economic activity in Britain in the years of great industrial and urban expansion in the eighteenth and nineteenth centuries, and more generally, the emergence of the medical profession was part of the wider rise of the middle classes in this period.[11] This is a large concept, but it is worth keeping in mind that Scottish medical societies, while distinct in nature and of intrinsic interest, were also part of a more general historical process.

The formation of professional societies is not an end in itself, however, as recognised by Noel and José Parry writing in 1976,

> We regard professionalism as an occupational strategy which is chiefly directed towards the achievement of upward collective social mobility and, once achieved, it is concerned with the maintenance of superior remuneration and status.[12]

The achievement and subsequent sustenance of enhanced status is a continuing thread in the history of professional medical development in Scotland and will be raised at various stages in this book. Again, the role of the 'formal association' is clear.

> The most strategic and treasured characteristic of the profession [is] ... its autonomy.... And the autonomy of the individual practitioner exists within the social and political space cleared and maintained for his benefit by political and occupational mechanisms.[13]

Another useful definition of a 'profession' since it is placed in an historical context and elaborates the nature of the 'common bonds' between the members of a profession, is contained in Geoffrey Holmes' study of professions in Augustan England.

> ... what gives it its distinctive social stamp is the fact that, through education and career-oriented training, a particular body of specialised knowledge is acquired and is then applied to the service (or it may be, the instruction or command) of others.... The assumption that this is usually expressed within some kind of institutional framework, and often under the auspices of some professional organisation or association with a supervising and regulating function must be almost as widespread. Such concepts as these were not alien to the 17th or early 18th century Englishman.[14]

This general description is particularly appropriate since it covers the late seventeenth and early eighteenth centuries. However, in relation to the practice of medicine, Holmes' subsequent assertion, ' ... it is between the years 1660 and 1740 that "the doctor" truly arrives in English society',[15] is the subject of debate given the traditional view of the evolution of the medical profession, which attributes the starting point of such a process to a much later date. 'In 1660 a physician was a gentleman, while apothecaries and surgeons were mere craftsmen; by 1800 it is possible to see them all as part of the new professional classes.'[16] Even for historians of more modern periods, such as Ivan Waddington, the eighteenth century is a period when medical practice was far from being a unified profession.

> It is important to remind ourselves, ... that throughout the 18th century, medicine not only had few of the characteristics which we associate with modern professions but that, even more basically, it was frequently not even a full-time occupation.[17]

Such a view is contested by Irvine Loudon, who sees many of the trends leading towards the elevation of medical practice to that of a profession well in evidence, if not in the period 1680–1730 as Holmes suggests, then certainly from 1740 onwards.[18] Such open debate on the timescale involved in the emergence of medicine as a profession is an indication of the complexities of this topic, particularly when the differences in professional development north and south of the border are considered in Chapter Three.

The main purpose of the first chapter is to provide an overview and outline of the main trends and developments in the history of the 160[19] Scottish medical societies in this survey from the point of view of the societies themselves, leaving the more detailed analysis of individual societies and their wider role in professional development to a later stage. The 135[20] senior medical societies had various functions, used different names, and had chequered histories: some lasted two years, others two centuries. Some societies had no obvious titular link with medicine, for example, convivial medical groups such as the Gymnastic Society[21] and the Round Table Club[22] which were set up in Edinburgh in the later eighteenth and nineteenth centuries respectively. Other societies are included even though their titles would suggest that they were not medical societies, for example the Edinburgh and Aberdeen Philosophical Societies. On closer examination however, it is clear that these two eighteenth century societies originally included many medical men and their discussions were originally dominated by scientific medical discussion.[23] The eighteenth-century Glasgow Philosophical Society by contrast did not include many medical practitioners or medical discussions,[24] and as such is not included in this survey. Other organisations with the misleading title of 'medical society' have not been included. For example, the Rutherglen Medical Society which existed in Glasgow in the 1920s, was a clinical medical centre staffed by local practitioners.[25] The nine phrenological societies in the survey represent only those societies with a prominent medical membership: numerous other phrenological societies with no such professional medical connection have been left out.

The role of the medical societies in the development of the medical profession is a vital one. Medical societies pursued (and continue to pursue) a variety of objectives. The various society types I have created in Chapter One are used to illuminate developments within the profession. For example, the close connection between the rise of medical scientific debate and the wider scientific and cultural advance of Edinburgh during the Scottish Enlightenment may be seen in the emergence of the early 'medico-scientific' societies. In the later nineteenth and early twentieth centuries, the rise of specialist disciplines such as paediatrics, can be measured by the creation of new, often exclusive, 'Scottish specialist societies'. After the gradual rise of medical societies in the eighteenth century, societies of various types grew in number throughout the nineteenth and early twentieth centuries, with few decades when the number of societies failing was not outstripped by the creation of new ones. This pattern of rise and fall is also traced in Chapter One.

A great variety of medical issues were discussed in the dozens of societies which existed in Scotland at various times. These issues have been categorised in Chapter Two to allow an overview of medical societies' functions. Throughout the period surveyed, the educational activities of medical societies, large and small, city or rural-based, remained important. Indeed, for many qualified practitioners membership of the local medical society (or societies) was the chief means of post-graduate education for the best part of two centuries down to the beginning of the twentieth century, when formal post-graduate courses were organised in Scottish hospitals.

Due in some measure to the success of Scottish University medical teaching, pressures on the expanding medical community increased in the course of the nineteenth century, when competition for patients and intra-professional rivalry for official appointments, combined with the numerical superiority of unlicensed practitioners, made the practice of medicine an uncertain and sometimes unrewarding profession. The precarious position of rank and file practitioners at this time helps to explain why the fixing of local fee structures and the attempted regulation of internal professional disputes, as described in Chapter Two, were major concerns for Scottish medical societies throughout the nineteenth century.

Competition for patients and competition for government posts was a characteristic of nineteenth-century medical society activity, yet clubs and societies also often had a strong social element. The convivial aspects of medical societies date back to the first societies established in Edinburgh in the second half of the eighteenth century, and while this more recreational function can sometimes appear to be of lesser importance than the educational and medico-political objects of society activity, it had a prominent role to play in bringing medical practitioners together in a convivial atmosphere. The social side of society activity could also provide an opportunity for a 'hidden agenda' of informal discussions between society members about the local profession in regard to hospital and government appointments in the area, and the rise of political factions. Such matters are rarely mentioned in society minutes, but are topics which would undoubtedly arise as members of a common profession gathered together.

The role of medical societies in local public health provision is an area which reveals the profession's role in the voluntary sector of welfare services. Society members' involvement in public health could range from the provision of free vaccination services, to the education and certification of local midwives, to financial support for medical missions, to taking the initiative in campaigns for the increase in local hospital provision.

The field of obstetrics provides an example of the ways in which a specific interest and related developments in therapeutics and medical science were addressed within the ranks of Scottish medical societies over a long period of time. The second chapter ends with a brief consideration of medical science and medico-scientific societies, and of society links with the international medical community.

In the eighteenth century, societies were initiated chiefly for the purposes of medical education, not only of their own members, but of the profession as a whole through the publication of transactions which often appeared in translation on the Continent, enabling Scottish societies and their discussions to reach, and to interact with the international medical community. Other objectives, such as the development of intra-professional cooperation also led to the setting up of the first Scottish medical societies and clubs. As will be shown in Chapter Three, almost all of the early societies were based in Edinburgh, reflecting the dominance of the University's medical school, although contributions to society transactions came from all over Scotland. The central role of medical societies in the history of Scottish medicine and professional development is emphasised by the close links between early medical societies and the medical faculties of the Scottish Universities. General practitioners inspired later societies.

The history of medical science and the development of the medical profession was not simply one of direct progression. Dubious methods of undertaking medical research and contentious areas of medical science were advocated. In these areas, tacit medical support and involvement in 'resurrectionism', and professional endorsement of phrenology will be considered in some detail in Chapter Four.

In Chapter Five the impact of government legislation on the Scottish medical profession will be assessed through the debates of Scottish medical societies; and in this respect the relationship between local societies as pressure groups and the emergence of the British Medical Association as the official 'political voice' of the profession is important. The far-reaching effects of the rise of 'state medicine' is a crucial element in professional development in the first decades of this century.

Other issues too, wrought great changes in the ranks of the medical profession. The rise of female practitioners and their fight for recognition within the profession for example, are to be found in the discussions of Scottish medical societies, particularly when their often unsuccessful attempts for admission to the ranks of local societies led to the setting up of their own medical societies.

The place of medical societies in the post Second World War, post-NHS, period will also be examined in a brief epilogue with reference to the enduring distinction between medical social clubs; exclusive scientific specialist societies; and the 'general interest' societies, which enjoy continued good health.

NOTES

1. *Medical Essays* (1732), pp. xix-xx.
2. Garioch and Northern Medical Association minute book, 4 May 1889, Aberdeen University Library Manuscripts Collection.
3. Medico-Chirurgical Society of Glasgow minute book, 2 December 1892, Royal College of Physicians and Surgeons Library, Glasgow.
4. Dundee Clinical Club, minute book 21 February 1903, Dundee University Archives.
5. Chronological lists of the 135 senior and 25 student and graduate medical societies are given in Appendices I and 2.
6. There are numerous articles which examine the importance of medical societies from a general (English) medical historical standpoint : Batty Shaw 'The Oldest Medical Societies' (1967), 232-44; Bishop, 'Medical Societies' (1950), 207-9; Bishop, 'Medical Book Societies' (1957), 337-50; Marland, 'Early 19th Century Medical Society Activity' (1985), 37-48; Rolleston, 'Medical Friendships' (1930), 249-66; Swan, 'Role and Position of Medical Societies' (1982), 43-7. See also Thornton (1949), ch. on 'The Rise of the Medical Societies', 130-44; and Hurry (1913); McMenemy, 'Influence of Medical Societies' ch. in Poynter (1961), mentions only one Scottish society. The best recent discussion of the role of English medical societies and associations can be found in Loudon (1986), *passim*.
7. There are a great number of articles and many books on individual Scottish societies, and these references are given under specific society entries in Part Two of this work.
8. Carr-Saunders and Wilson (1930), 298.
9. *Ibid.*, 295.
10. *Ibid.*, 327.
11. Peterson (1979), 1.
12. N. and J. Parry (1976), 79.
13. Friedson (1972), pp. 23-4.
14. Holmes (1982), 3.
15. *Ibid.*, 167.
16. Hamilton, 'Medical Profession in the 18th century' (1951), 141.
17. Waddington (1984), 189.
18. Loudon (1986), pp. 12-13 *passim*.
19. See Appendices 1 and 2 for chronological lists of the senior and student and graduate medical societies surveyed.
20. The 25 student and graduate medical societies in Scotland during these years are listed separately in Appendix 2, but will be discussed from time to time in the course of this work.
21. See Part Two entry 87 for more specific information on the Gymnastic Society.
22. See Part Two entry 48 for more on the Round Table Club. For subsequent cited medical societies refer to Part Two of this book, where information on individual societies is listed in alphabetical order.
23. See Emerson's series of articles on 'Philosophical Society of Edinburgh' (1979), 154-91; (1981), 133-76; (1985), 255-303; (1988), 33-66. For the Aberdeen Philosophical Society see Ulman (1990), *passim*.
24. Membership of the Glasgow Philosophical Society, established in 1802, more than 60 years after the Edinburgh Philosophical and almost 50 years after the Aberdeen Philosophical, was chiefly made up of manufacturers, artisans and merchants, see Morrell 'Reflections on the History of Scottish Science' (1974), 80.
25. See minute book of the Glasgow Southern Medical Society 11 November 1926, Victoria Infirmary Library, Glasgow.

CHAPTER ONE

Scottish Medical Societies 1731–1939: Their Number and Organisation

TYPES OF MEDICAL SOCIETY

Seven society types were created to lay down a structure for the better assessment of the 135 senior societies included in this survey.[1] These are:

'general interest' medical societies: open to all qualified practitioners

'convivial' societies, i.e. dining or social groupings

medico-scientific, general scientific and philosophical societies: these latter two groups were originally dominated by medical men and interests but later became more general in their scientific and philosophic concerns

medical-related societies: a grouping which includes medical missionary societies and lay organisations with a strong interest for the profession, e.g. the Edinburgh Health Society

'single discipline' societies: devoted to a specific branch or aspect of medicine but open to all medical practitioners

'Scottish specialist' societies: Scotland-wide organisations open only to those practising in the field

'professional protection' organisations: medical defence associations and medical occupational interest groups

The largest and most wide ranging type defined is the 'general interest' medical society. Sixty-three (46 per cent) of the societies come under this category. A 'general interest' medical society is one which is open to all qualified medical practitioners.[2] Any branch of medicine and medical science could be considered for discussion by the members. Medical politics and matters of professional etiquette could also on occasion be raised. Within this wide ranging society type some characteristics were more common than others. Not every society had a permanent meeting place; some of the smaller, and/or shorter-lived societies met in rotation in members' houses, while other societies rented rooms in coffee houses or public halls. Similarly, not every society possessed its own library, although the informal circulation of books or medical journals may have taken place between members of societies without such facilities. All societies did however, by their nature contain some kind of social element, and it would be true to say that this became more formalised as the society developed in size and organisation (annual dinners were, and continue to be, the chief form of such occasions).

Other medical societies and clubs were expressly created for the purpose of developing social contacts between members of the profession, and these form the second type of society devised. The setting up of convivial societies demonstrated a common interest and outlook which, even if it did not stretch beyond sharing a meal together, is important since it provides evidence of the growing professional links between practitioners. It dated from the late eighteenth century when the first of the Scottish medical social clubs began to emerge. The Aesculapian Club established in Edinburgh in 1773 is the first example of this primarily social grouping, although even in this type of society pressures could still be brought to bear on disputatious members in the interest of the profession as a whole.[3]

The third society type, medico-scientific and general scientific and philosophical societies,[4] played a prominent part in the development of the medical profession in Scotland from the mid-eighteenth century until well into the nineteenth century, and Edinburgh was the centre of this type of society activity.[5]

> It is to the credit of our two Royal Colleges [of Physicians and Surgeons respectively] that those of their members who were to form in 1821 the Medico-Chirurgical Society had previously furnished so many office-bearers to the scientific societies which then served to connect medicine with general science.[6]

The fourth category encompasses medical-related societies, for example, those which dealt with an issue of strong medical interest, but were open to lay people e.g. the Edinburgh Health Society; and the charity-based medical missionary societies. The first Scottish medical missionary society, the Edinburgh Medical Missionary Society, set up in 1841, was originally intended solely to train medical students to undertake missionary work for the Church of Scotland overseas, but after 1853 its work, and that of subsequent medical missions, was expanded to include the provision of free dispensaries and attendance on the poor in the local community. Other medical missions were established in Glasgow, Aberdeen and Inverness in the 1860s, and their activities serve as a reminder that the medical profession was part of the wider community, and that medical practitioners became active, like so many of their mid-Victorian counterparts, in philanthropic endeavour.

The three remaining types of medical society are: those devoted to a single medical discipline but open to all practitioners during the period in question; Scottish 'specialist' societies formed to provide a forum for specialists in a distinct field of medicine; and 'professional protection' societies such as the Scottish Medical Defence Association, and the Scottish Poor Law Medical

Officers' Association. These three types are relatively modern inventions, and they reflect the diversified nature of Scottish medical societies in the later nineteenth and early twentieth centuries.

The Ascent

The success of the Scottish Universities' system of medical education after 1730 created an expanding sector of educated medical men who practised alongside empirics or 'quacks', as the contemporary 'qualified' profession viewed their 'unqualified' competitors for the nation's health care.[7] In the late eighteenth century and increasingly in the first half of the nineteenth century, these groups came into direct competition, and on occasion, conflict, as they sought to earn a living. This situation made some method of ensuring cooperation, minimising intra-professional rivalry, agreeing fee levels, and improving the status of the 'qualified' rank and file practitioner a necessity. That the medical profession formed medical societies when faced with this increasing threat to their livelihood owed much to the influence and example of the medical elite of the eighteenth century Scottish Enlightenment.

For much of the eighteenth century the focus of professional organisation was on Edinburgh where the first attempts at association were directed at overcoming the divisions between the separate medical corporations of physicians and surgeons.[8] As medical societies achieved a wider geographical spread around the country by the early nineteenth century the emphasis came to be on providing an alternative to this rather exclusive hierarchy of the medical corporations, which represented the interests of the elite level of medical practitioners[9] by seeking to perpetuate a geographical as well as status-related closed shop at the same time as excluding the 'irregular' practitioners.

The first Scottish medical society was the Edinburgh Medical Society, set up in 1731, five years after the formation of the medical faculty of the University of Edinburgh in 1726, and only two years after the opening of the first voluntary hospital in Scotland, the Edinburgh Hospital for the Sick Poor (which became the Royal Infirmary after 1736). These two events provided the dynamic for the new, albeit relatively short-lived, society whose published transactions included many contributions from the professoriate of the recently created medical faculty of Edinburgh University.

> When patients were received into the infirmary, and a regular register kept of all their cases, it was reasonably expected that many histories worth publishing might be extracted from that register, and might assist to form volumes of medical observations or essays, which it was proposed should be published from time to time. With this view, the professors of physic associated with Drs Drummond senior, Francis Pringle, Lewis, Clerk, Cochran, Porterfield, Dundas, and Mr MacGill, surgeon [to form a society]. Professor Monro was appointed their secretary...[10]

The Edinburgh Medical Society lasted only until 1737, but its creation and purpose (to disseminate medical knowledge and facilitate clinical and scientific discussion) was an indication of a new trend in Scottish medical practice, centred in Edinburgh, in which education through association became the key. The creation of the 'student' Royal Medical Society of Edinburgh[11] was also closely linked to the rapid rise of the medical faculty of the University and may also have owed more than a little to the influence of the Edinburgh Medical Society:

> In the autumn of 1734 six students of medicine *fired by the example of their masters* [my emphasis] who had nothing more at heart than the improvement of those who committed themselves to their tuition, began to hold informal meetings for the discussion of dissertations, written by themselves, on medical subjects. This little association laid the foundation of the Medical Society in 1737...[12]

The formation and characteristics of many of the eighteenth–century student medical societies echoed that of their senior counterparts in a period when many of the 'students' drawn to Edinburgh were already in practice and had come to the University to augment their medical education. The creation of the Royal Medical Society set the pattern for eighteenth century Scottish student societies, 83 per cent of which were based in Edinburgh (see Appendix 2). The setting up of the Aberdeen Medical (later Medico-Chirurgical) Society in 1789 demonstrates how strong an influence was the example provided by the Edinburgh student societies.

> The prime movers in the foundation of the new society were James McGrigor and his companion, James Robertson, who at the completion of their studies at Marischal College, had proceeded to Edinburgh to study under Monro secundus, and while there had attended meetings of similar students' societies.[13]

The general numerical and geographical supremacy of Edinburgh, in both senior and student medical societies was challenged only towards the end of the eighteenth century by Aberdeen and Glasgow, whose newly created student societies in the former and convivial club in the latter, were based on the model of the Edinburgh clubs and societies (see Appendices 1 and 2 and Figures 1.1 and 1.2). A more general point is that medical science and education were part of the wider scientific and cultural milieu of Edinburgh elite society in this period of the 'Scottish Enlightenment'.[14] The influence of this wider cultural development may be denoted by the fact that of the 11 medical and medical-related societies[15] established in Scotland between 1731 and 1799 only three were 'general interest' medical societies, while 4 were medically-dominated scientific or philosophical groupings and a further 4 were convivial clubs. Eight of the 11 societies in question were set up in Edinburgh.

An indication of how far the setting up of a society had come to be the recognised manner of demonstrating scientific or cultural merit during the Scottish Enlightenment may be taken by reference to the creation of a fictitious

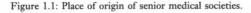
Figure 1.1: Place of origin of senior medical societies.

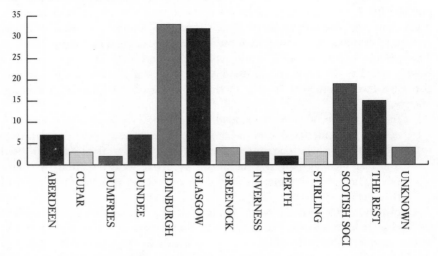

Figure 1.2: Place of origin of student and graduate societies.

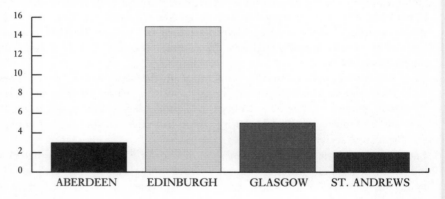

publishing society by Andrew Duncan senior (then an extra-mural lecturer in medicine in Edinburgh, after 1789, Professor of the Institutes of Medicine at Edinburgh University). Duncan attributed the work included in his *Medical and Philosophical Commentaries* to that of a fictitious medical society to associate his *Commentaries* with the successful tradition of society transactions: epitomised by those of the Edinburgh Medical Society and its successor, the Edinburgh Philosophical Society:

> In 1771, when a new publication was undertaken under the title of *Medical and Philosophical Commentaries*, ... it was an established custom for such publications to be the work of a society. In keeping with the tradition, it was announced on the title page of the new publication that it was 'by a Society in Edinburgh'. This 'Society' however, never existed, despite

those who have claimed the contrary... only one man was really responsible... Andrew Duncan.[16]

The *Commentaries* were the precursor of the long-lived *Edinburgh Medical
Journal* (originally the *Edinburgh Medical and Surgical Journal*), which gave
much prominence to the activities of medical societies.

In addition to his interest in the publication of medical periodicals, Duncan
senior was the leading figure behind the creation of several leading medical clubs
and societies in Edinburgh, including the Aesculapian Club, and the Harveian,
Gymnastic, and the Edinburgh Medico-Chirurgical Societies. Despite what has
proved to be the considerable longevity of three of these groups, Duncan was
not without his contemporary critics:

> He was a kind-hearted and excellent man; but one of a class which seems
> to live and be happy, and get liked, by its mere absurdities. He was the
> promoter and the president of more innocent and foolish clubs and
> societies than perhaps any man in the world...[17]

Educational improvement achieved through association and publication was
important in the development of the medical profession in Scotland, particularly
Edinburgh, after the 1730s, but other factors also helped facilitate the notion of a
medical 'community'. Between 1760 and 1800 at least six[18] medical social clubs
were established in the city, of which the best known are: the Aesculapian Club;
the Harveian Society; and the Gymnastic Society. Under the auspices of
Duncan senior, these three bodies sought to bring medical practitioners together
(both physicians and surgeons who belonged to separate corporations in the city)
in an atmosphere of fraternity and sociability. The social aspect of medical
societies dominant in these three organisations came to play an integral part in
all medical societies after this period. Reference to the Aesculapian Club
provides a clear example of the role of medical societies and clubs in creating a
focus for developing professional relationships, since it was from its inception
open to equal numbers of physicians and surgeons.

> The main object of the Club, which has been fully realised, was, to cement
> the friendship between the Two Royal Colleges, of Physicians and Sur-
> geons. Accordingly, the first regulation reads: 'The Club shall consist of
> twenty-two members, chosen from among the Fellows of the Colleges of
> Physicians and Surgeons'.[19]

The issue of professional cooperation and matters of ethical behaviour (medical
etiquette) is also important in the study of the development of the medical
profession dating from the eighteenth century, as is the role of medical societies
in providing a forum for regulating relationships between medical practitioners.[20]
However, at this early stage of the discussion it would be wrong other than to
signal this as a factor in the rise of medical societies. Concern for the regulation
of matters of professional etiquette does however, provide a link between the
eighteenth- and nineteenth-century societies, and is part of the more general
tendency of the early nineteenth-century societies towards the 'professional
improvement' of their members. This phrase was often a keynote in a society's

own definition of its aims in the early nineteenth century, as an extract from a letter by J. Inglis Nicol, an Inverness surgeon, to the *Edinburgh Medical and Surgical Journal*[21] in 1821 aptly demonstrates:

> From the interest you take in everything that tends to improve our profession, I am sure you will be pleased to hear that an association has been formed in the capital of the Highlands, under the designation of the Medical Society of the North, *whose objects are the improvement of the profession in all its departments* [my emphasis]. This society, which now consists of upwards of 30 members, was formed in 1817, but intimation was withheld until we saw how it prospered.[22]

This phrase appears again in the announcement of the creation of the Fifeshire Medico-Chirurgical Society in 1826, a year after its formation:

> The Professional gentlemen of the county of Fife have united themselves into a Medico-Chirurgical Society which is to hold meetings at stated times for mutual improvement, and the communication of professional knowledge.[23]

As well as a perceptible change in emphasis in these early nineteenth-century societies away from the wider cultural concerns and towards 'professional' issues, there was also an expanded geographical spread of medical societies and clubs around the country (See Figure 1.1). Whereas Edinburgh medical societies dominated in the second half of the eighteenth century, tied to the rise of the medical faculty and its clinical teaching in the Royal Infirmary, the period between 1805 and 1840 was one in which medical societies and clubs were established in Inverness, Greenock, Paisley, Dumfries, Dundee, Cupar (Fife), Kilmarnock, Forfar, Stirling, Clackmannan, Kelso (the Borders), and Perth (see Appendix 1).

The spread of medical societies around the country suggests a growth in the number of 'qualified' practitioners who felt a common bond and recognised the benefits of association in order to protect their livelihood and enhance their status. The continued success of the Edinburgh medical school and the development of the Glasgow medical faculty helps account for the increase in the number of 'qualified' practitioners indicated by the setting up of societies in areas which were by no means large centres of population,[24] and yet apparently contained enough medical practitioners in close proximity to allow a society to be established. The influence of example of the many student medical societies in Edinburgh, the student Medical Society in Aberdeen and the Glasgow University Medico-Chirurgical Society[25] (1802) to which many local practitioners would have belonged during their days at University, may also be a factor in the spread of societies. The increase in the number of 'qualified' practitioners also owes something to the change in status of the medical profession in Scotland wrought during the second part of the eighteenth century, since medicine was becoming a more attractive profession for the middle classes.[26]

Increases in the numbers of practitioners also brought increased competition for patients; consequently a new emphasis on the fixing of local fees and more

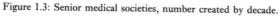

Figure 1.3: Senior medical societies, number created by decade.

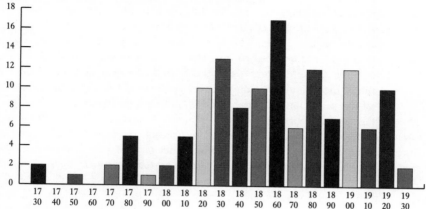

general medico-political matters was apparent in society activity in the early nineteenth century. Particularly after 1815, Scottish medical societies displayed a keen interest in medico-political matters as campaigns for the reform of medical education and for the recognition of 'legally qualified' practitioners became of increasing importance in an expanding medical sector numerically dominated by those without professional qualifications of any kind. The 1830s, when thirteen medical societies were set up, was a particularly active period in medico-political discussion. This decade in fact, saw the highest number of societies established in a decade until the 1860s (see Figure 1.3).

The campaign for the reform of medical education is perhaps the most well-known aspect of national medical societies, and local Scottish societies were part of the national campaign to press the government into action on behalf of the profession throughout the nineteenth century. The 1815 Apothecaries' Act, which had given legal definition to the term 'medically qualified', also had the negative effect of forcing Scottish, Irish, and foreign medical graduates who wanted to practice in England, to undergo a further five years' apprenticeship to enable them to sit for a licence in the Apothecaries' Hall, after 1815, a necessary qualification for legal practice in England. In part due to such anomalies, cumulative pressures brought to bear by medical societies throughout the British Isles helped to facilitate the introduction of seventeen medical bills in the years from 1840 down to the eventual passage of the Medical Act of 1858. A public meeting in Stirling in June 1840 to draw up a petition to Parliament in favour of medical reform highlighted the pressure group activities of several of the Scottish medical societies,

> The object of the present meeting is ... to consider the subject of medical reform.... Numerous associations of medical practitioners have been formed for the purpose of promoting it. Amongst these, the British Medical Association, (the original Association, unrelated to the present BMA which was initially known as the Provincial Medical and Surgical

Association, see below), the Irish Medical Association, the Provincial Medical Association of England, (sic), itself composed of at least 1200 members, and the Eastern and Western Medical Associations of Scotland, hold conspicuous places. The Committee of the Stirling Medical Association, an institution formed for other purposes than those of medical reform, have also deemed it expedient, in the present position of matters, to solicit the opinion, not only of the members of this association, but also of all the practitioners in the district, on this important subject.[27]

The various medical bills laid before Parliament between 1840 and 1858 sought to end unregulated medical practice and to organise national medical education. But, owing in large part to the negative influence of the ancient, well-established medical corporations acting as a group with a vested interest in maintaining the status quo, it was eighteen years before even a measure as limited as the 1858 Act was able to gain sufficient support to be enacted. This Act has been regarded as a crucial turning point in the history of the medical profession in Britain.

The 1858 Medical Act is generally regarded as a major legislative landmark – perhaps the major legislative landmark – in the development of the medical profession, for in establishing the General Medical Council and in requiring the Council to maintain a register of all qualified practitioners the Act established an important part of the institutional framework of the modern medical profession in Britain.[28]

A more convincing assessment of the 1858 Act is provided by Loudon,

it is sometimes suggested that, for all its failings, at least the Medical Act was responsible for unifying the profession; but this is nonsense, confusing causes with results. The Medical Act of 1858, like the Apothecaries Act of 1815 was the product, not the cause of changes in the profession.[29]

The Medical Act of 1858, although it did not go as far as medical reformers, including the increasing number of medical societies with medico-political interests, would have liked in outlawing 'unqualified' medical practice, made provision for a system of national registration of 'qualified' practitioners. This recognition in turn increased the social cache of medical society membership as a form of common identification for the profession, since all societies made the possession of a medical qualification an essential prerequisite for entry.

The desire for identification with the 'organised' profession can be put forward in partial explanation for the sudden growth in the number of Scottish medical societies in the ten years which followed the passage of the 1858 Act. Seventeen of the 135 Scottish societies identified to date, or 13 per cent of the total, were formed in the 1860s (see Figure 1.3). Moreover, the decade after 1858 saw not only a great numerical increase among Scottish medical societies, but a trend towards more formalised, visible, associations of medical practitioners, as the official recognition of the profession was now a matter of printed record in the shape of the *Medical Register*. Information on societies established in the 1860s is more readily available to the researcher in the form of surviving records, reports of their activities in the medical press, and entries in the *Medical Directory*, than similar information on associations of, for example, the 1830s (mentioned earlier as the second most important period for medical society establishment, when thirteen societies (10 per cent) are recorded as being set up). Despite the increasing number and visibility of societies in the 1860s, there are few changes in the structure and motives of the newer organisations, than with their 1830s counterparts. Basic medical society functions such as the possession of a library and specimens, discussion on matters of local professional regulation, fee-fixing, and medical politics, and the holding of dinners and other social events, are common to both periods. Neither do societies in the earlier period seem more transient than those of the 1860s.

Of the 8 medical societies set up in the 1860s whose date of cessation has been established, 3 lasted ten years or less. Exact dates of cessation are known for only 4 of the 13 societies formed in the 1830s, the shortest-lived society lasted twelve years; however it is probable that some of the other societies, particularly the phrenological societies, had relatively brief life-spans. Of course, the lack of complete data in this area weakens the impact of this point, but there is enough evidence to suggest that the greatly increased number of societies established in the 1860s could not be sustained by the medical community in Scotland for any length of time, particularly bearing in mind that there were 23 medical and related scientific societies already in existence by this time.

Eight of the 17 societies formed in the decade 1860-70 were set up in the geographical area stretching from Dundee northwards, a figure out of proportion when the overall geographical balance of Scottish medical societies is considered (see Figure 1.1). The general factors affecting the practice of medicine in Scotland as a whole no doubt affected the northern part of the country also, but the great growth in the number of northern Scottish societies formed at this time may also have been due to improvements in transport in the course of the century which allowed more ready communication between medical practitioners in the area. In addition, there was more of a market for medical associations in a region which could boast only 3 of the 23 medical and related associations in existence before 1860.

The passing of the Medical Act of 1858 discussed earlier does seem to have had a positive effect on the regard for medical societies among the profession in general. The success achieved (albeit limited) by the existing medical societies in speeding the passage of the 1858 Act also served as an example of what could be attained in terms of legislation by medical pressure groups, and this again helped to promote the cause of the medical society as an institution in the 1860s. Indeed, the creation of two of the three societies set up in the years 1858-9 can be directly attributed to the passage of the 1858 Act. The Forfarshire Medical Association and the Association of Scottish Medical Practitioners were both established to help implement the clauses of the Act. The Forfarshire Medical Association was: 'formed to assist the working of the New Medical Act, and to take a general supervision of medical affairs in the county of Forfar'.[30] While the

Scottish Association of Medical Practitioners was established in February 1859 after '... a meeting of the Registered Medical Practitioners of Scotland was held at Edinburgh, in the Royal Hotel, for the purpose of forming an Association to promote the enforcement of the Medical Act'.[31]

The formation of the Association of Scottish Medical Practitioners was the first attempt at a 'professional protection'[32] society in Scotland. It was the intention of the Association to use the ten shilling membership fee from members as a legal fund in order to prosecute unregistered practitioners in the courts. The Association was however, short-lived in consequence of the Procurator Fiscal's refusal to undertake such prosecutions, which were not within the scope of the 1858 Medical Act.[33] This move towards a country-wide Scottish organisation of medical practitioners, however transient, is worth noting here, as it foreshadows a trend in national organisation which influenced the response of local Scottish societies to the expansion of regional branches of the British Medical Association to Scotland.[34]

Due to a combination of circumstances, Edinburgh was the centre of medical society creation in the eighteenth century. By the first half of the nineteenth century, however, societies were set up across Scotland. Overall, the period 1830–70 was the most vigorous one in the history of Scottish medical societies. Forty-eight societies were established during these years (see Figure 1.3) and within this period, the twenty year span from 1850–70 saw an average 1.4 societies created each year. Could this growth rate be sustained?

The Descent

It is difficult to trace a comparable pattern for the decline in medical societies and to relate this to the wider context of the professional trends, since information is rarely given on why societies failed. Minute book entries in failing societies most often come to an abrupt end, with little to forewarn the reader other than a decline in the regularity of meetings convened. However, several general causes in the termination of medical societies such as the decline in member interest, insufficient funds, and the death of motivating members, have been identified. Looking beyond this, a detailed analysis of the figures provided recording the demise of societies is problematic since of the 135 societies listed, the date of cessation of 51 (38 per cent) is unknown or not certain (see Appendix 1). Of the remainder, 33 (24 per cent) are currently in existence, while a further 51 (38 per cent) do have attributable dates of cessation.

Looking at the 51 societies whose date of cessation is known, it is immediately clear that there is not enough information on the exact end date of societies to create the same type of analysis as was carried out for the rise of societies (see Figure 1.4). Having said this, there are two decades which stand out as times when medical societies fortunes do appear to have declined; in the 1870s and 1930s when seven societies disappeared in the course of each decade: this figure was considerably higher than the average failure rate of 3 per decade which was displayed in the period from the 1800 to the 1930s, (only 3 societies are known

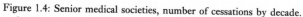

Figure 1.4: Senior medical societies, number of cessations by decade.

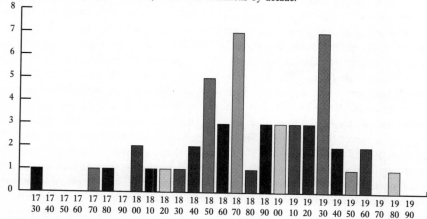

to have failed in the years between 1731 and 1799, and 6 since 1940, hence the exclusion of these periods from the calculations). Looking at the decade 1870–80 in detail, 4 of the 7 societies which ceased in this period had been established only in the previous 'boom' decade, but this fact should not be regarded as too meaningful, since a further 5 of the 1860s societies lasted until well into the twentieth century, including the Royal Odonto-Chirurgical Society of Scotland, which is still in existence.

The other notable decade for the demise of Scottish medical societies is 1930–40. Of the 7 societies which came to an end in this decade 5 failed between 1931–5 (the other 2 coming to an end with the outbreak of war in 1939), which perhaps suggests that if any underlying cause other than the death of members, were to account for this fact, then the depressed economic situation of the country as a whole was forcing medical practitioners to restrain their expenditure levels at a time when the membership of a medical society may have been regarded as an expendable luxury.

The durability of Scottish medical societies in general is worth commenting on: although 11 of the 135 societies analysed are known to have lasted less than ten years, 20 have lasted more than a century, and 5 of these have existed for more than 200 years[35] (see Appendix 1). Such figures suggest that while medical societies were open to the wider influence of the state of the medical profession as a whole, (and perhaps, of completely external factors, such as the national economy), they also possessed an internal dynamic and localised dimension, and it was these latter two factors which, ultimately, accounted for their continued success or failure.

THE ADVANCE OF MEDICAL SPECIALITY AND THE ECLIPSE OF 'GENERAL INTEREST' MEDICAL SOCIETIES

Throughout this chapter the intention has been to outline the variety of forms manifested by medical and related societies, and to chart their varying fortunes.

The seven society types have been described, and the 'general interest' medical society, open to all practitioners, mentioned as the largest group of all the medical societies surveyed. The final three society types; the 'single discipline'; 'Scottish specialist' societies; and the 'professional protection' organisations; collectively account for 20 per cent of the sample. This is a relatively high figure, particularly considering that all the societies in these groups were established after 1839, and thus within the last hundred years of a 240-year time scale. There is however, a major difference between the categories: the 'single discipline' societies, dealing with a particular branch or aspect of medicine or medical science, unlike their 'Scottish specialist' counterparts, were open to general practitioners and did not restrict their membership only to those pursuing a medical career within the field of medicine they represented. The 'professional protection' associations ranged from those intent on representing the professional interests of the whole profession, to those out to safeguard the position of a limited group of practitioners employed by the state. Thus, these three categories must be examined as separate entities.

The first 'single discipline' society in Scotland was the Edinburgh Obstetrical Society[36] established in 1840. From its outset it was a society open to general practitioners who practised midwifery. Indeed, it remained as such until after the Second World War as obstetrics continued to play an integral part of day-to-day general practice. Some later nineteenth-century 'single discipline' societies also sought a broader base than is suggested by their title, as an account of the formation of the Edinburgh Pathological Club in 1886, reveals,

> In spite of its name the Pathological Club has been largely concerned with matters not strictly pathological. Those who founded the Club in a rapidly-growing atmosphere of specialism soon realised that, while it was essential to know as much as possible about one's own branch of medical learning, it was equally important to listen to the opinions and criticism of workers in other fields.[37]

The professionally-exclusive 'Scottish specialist' societies did not begin to emerge until the early twentieth century (see Appendix 1). The timing of their establishment is not surprising since it closely follows the emergence of a separate class of medical 'specialists' towards the end of the nineteenth century. The distinction must be made at this point between doctors who 'consulted' each other in certain difficult cases, or those individual practitioners who had acquired sufficient eminence to be actively sought by wealthy patients, practices which had a long history; and the much more recent evolution of 'pure consultants': specialists in a particular field of medicine, frequently hospital-based, to whom other practitioners referred patients. There were of course, earlier nineteenth-century 'part-time consultants' who continued to work as general practitioners to the wealthy while pursuing their specialist work, but it is safe to assume that their numbers were restricted until the end of the nineteenth century, and that competition rather than cooperation would be the determining factor in relations between those who did practise a speciality at this early stage.

The consultant was not even a specialist at first; rather he was by definition, a doctor called in by other doctors to give a second opinion. He was also in most cases, an honorary physician or surgeon at a voluntary hospital – an important element in the gradual transition of the consultant into the office-based specialist. As late as 1870 there were very few 'pure consultants' in the United Kingdom. Most of them were practising as general practitioners to the rich middle classes.[38]

The first 'Scottish specialist' society set up was the Scottish Otological and Laryngological Society in 1910. The Society held its inaugural meeting, attended by twenty-eight members, in Edinburgh Royal Infirmary in November 1910, at which it was decided that eligibility should be on the basis of holding a university, hospital or dispensary appointment in this 'special branch of medicine'.[39] Closer consideration of the 'Scottish specialist' societies allows a fairly clear pattern to emerge. Seven were formed in the period between 1910 and 1938 and they generally met in rotation at the four major University-based medical schools of the country at Edinburgh, Glasgow, Aberdeen and Dundee (St Andrews University) as there was an increasing overlap between academic and hospital consultant posts. For example, the Scottish Society for Experimental Medicine at its inception in 1938 included eight professors among its strictly limited membership of twenty-six.[40]

Of the final type of society, the 'professional protection' organisations, only those independent Scottish organisations have been included in this survey. National professional organisations which had branches in Scotland are not listed. Some of the Scottish organisations had British counterparts, and indeed, the Society of Medical Officers of Health for Scotland became a branch of the national Society of Medical Officers of Health in 1908, but at its creation in 1891, it was an independent body which met separately from the national organisation to defend the interests of Scottish Medical Officers of Health.

The rise of speciality and the subsequent pressure on the existence of general interest societies may help account for the failure of seven medical societies in the 1930s, six of which were 'general interest' societies. The increased failure rate for the local, 'general interest', medical society during the 1930s would mean little in itself, were it not for the fact that it closely followed a period, 1910–22, in which five 'Scottish specialist' societies had been set up, among them the Scottish Society of Anaesthetists in 1914, and the Scottish Paediatric Society in 1922. The rise of speciality in these years did not however, signal the end of vigorous all-practitioner activity in matters of pressing medical interest: single discipline societies also continued to be formed in this period, for example, the Tuberculosis Society of Scotland which was established in 1921 and was open to '... all persons qualified in medicine resident in Scotland.'[41] Also continuing to emerge in the early twentieth century period were 'professional protection' societies, such as the Association of School Medical Officers for Scotland established in 1911. Such societies, some of them dating from the later nineteenth century,[42] were set up to help forge a link across Scotland between those pursuing a part-time government sponsored medical occupation.

Changes in regard to the further education of the medical profession in Scotland further conspired to reduce the attraction of local 'general interest' societies in the early decades of the twentieth century. The introduction of post-graduate teaching in the medical faculties of Edinburgh and Glasgow Universities at the beginning of the twentieth century,[43] was soon augmented by post-graduate classes offered during the summer months by staff at the major hospitals. In 1912, for example, it was announced that, 'the Medical staff of the (Glasgow) Western Infirmary have arranged to conduct during September post-graduate courses in clinical medicine and the diseases of the skin.'[44] The following year courses were being offered at both the Glasgow Royal Infirmary and the Western, the latter making particular reference to the relevance of its courses for general practitioners, '... special attention will be directed to digestive disturbances, nervous diseases, gall-bladder disease, and the surgery of general practice'.[45] By 1928, the provision of post-graduate education for medical practitioners in Glasgow had come under the control of a central coordinating body.

A central organisation has been formed – the Glasgow Post-Graduate Medical Association – for the purpose of arranging, co-ordinating, and administering post-graduate medical education in Glasgow and the West of Scotland. General and special courses will be arranged and duly advertised. A comprehensive permanent scheme has been adopted. A special course for practitioners is held in the last fortnight of August and the first fortnight of September at the Royal and Victoria Infirmaries. Particulars may be obtained from Dr James Carslaw, The University.[46]

This development meant that after a period of almost 200 years one of the hitherto primary functions of the local 'general interest' medical societies: that of mutual education between those already engaged in the practice of medicine, began to be institutionalised and centrally-based.

An analysis of the 33 surviving Scottish medical societies established before 1939 suggests that the link established between the creation of 'Scottish specialist' societies and the decline of 'general interest' societies should not be overstated. Five of the current societies are 'Scottish specialist' organisations, but all of these are twentieth century institutions. Of the 13 remaining 'general interest' societies, all but 4 have lasted over a century, with an average life-span of 137 years. While speciality was becoming increasingly important within the Scottish medical profession in the early twentieth century, membership of well-established 'general interest' societies was still considered important, at a time when, with the increasing use of motor cars by the profession, access to the nearest large city and sizeable group of fellow practitioners became a relatively simple matter. It is no coincidence that of the 13 surviving 'general interest' medical societies from the pre-1939 period 5 are centred in Edinburgh, 4 in Glasgow, while Aberdeen, Dundee, Greenock and Paisley have one each.

The progress and concerns of local medical societies emphasise and illustrate the development of medicine as a profession in Scotland, in three key areas: the variety of medical societies and their fluctuating fortunes throughout the period; the link between medical societies and general professional development; and, how this helps to illustrate the increasing division between the general practitioner and the specialist from the beginning of the twentieth century. In examining these areas, stress has been placed on the constructive aspects of professional association in the local groups, but the less productive side must also be remembered. For example, as the profession's membership of phrenological societies shows, medical science was not a progressive upward spiral. At a personal level competition between individual practitioners led to petty jealousies and internal rivalries, making 'ethical' committees as much a necessity as a symbol of increasing professional awareness, and jeopardising the trend towards the enhanced status of the profession which was behind so much medical society activity. Yet such local rivalry was by no means confined to the province of medical societies. In reflecting the wider issues involved in the professionalisation of medicine, medical societies are consequential in their own right.

NOTES

1. See Appendix 1 for a chronological list of senior societies, with dates of existence and appropriate society-type code.
2. The exclusion of female medical practitioners by medical society members proved the exception to this rule until the beginning of the twentiethth century, see Chapter Five, pp. 93–7.
3. See Chapter Two, p. 34, for more on this dispute between fellow Aesculapians Professors Miller and Simpson in the mid-nineteenth century.
4. General scientific societies are included where the society had its origins in medical or medico-scientific investigation: the Royal Physical Society of Edinburgh set up in 1783 is an example of this type of society.
5. See Chapter Three, pp. 57–65, for more on the formation of medical societies and clubs in Edinburgh in the eighteenth century.
6. Handyside, 'Address to the Edinburgh Medico-Chirurgical Society' (1874), 770.
7. See Chapter Three, pp. 53–5, for a fuller discussion on the development of Scottish medical education and the attempt to exclude the unqualified from medical practice.
8. Many authors have addressed the role of Edinburgh medicine in the development of the Scottish Enlightenment, including Lawrence (1984), Shapin, 'Audience for Science in Eighteenth Century Edinburgh' (1974), 95-121, and Bynum and Porter (1985).
9. A discussion on the emergence of the elite profession in Edinburgh in the eighteenth century, despite continued divisions between the physicians' and surgeons' corporations appears in Chapter Three, pp. 53–7.
10. *Edinburgh Magazine and Review* April 1774, 339 quoted in McElroy (1952), 83.
11. For more on the activities of the Royal Medical Society, see Chapters Three and Four, pp. 63–5, 68–72.
12. Gray (1952), 2.
13. Craig, 'Aberdeen Medico-Chirurgical Society' (1968), 5.
14. See Chapter Three, pp. 59–63, for more on the history of Scottish medical development in this period.
15. The category of medical-related society is a problematical one, for there were many scientific societies established in Edinburgh in the eighteenth century. However, it is not always clear which of these had a prominent medical membership. Those included in this survey are ones for which I have either first-hand knowledge or reliable information as to the presence of medical practitioners in their ranks.
16. McElroy (1952), 471.

17. Cockburn (1910), 272.
18. There were at least three other medical social clubs established in Edinburgh during this period whose history is less well documented; The Dissipation Club is listed in Part Two of this book, while only the titles of the Galenian and Celsian societies have been identified, see McElroy (1952), pp. 312-3.
19. Guthrie 'Aesculapian Club' (1967), 245.
20. See Chapter Two, pp. 57–9, for more on the professional ethical concerns of medical societies.
21. This publication, directly descended from the *Medical Commentaries*, was edited for a time by Duncan and his son, also Andrew Duncan.
22 *Edinburgh Medical and Surgical Journal* 17 (1821), 317.
23. *EMSJ* 25 (1826), 241.
24. The rise of an industrial centre was a factor which could attract medical practitioners to an area.
25. For more on the Glasgow student medical society, see the student and graduate section of Part Two of this work.
26. Loudon (1986), 208.
27. *Stirling Journal and Advertiser*, 26 June 1840, 4.
28. Waddington (1984), 96.
29. Loudon (1986), 300.
30. *Medical Directory* (1861), 827.
31. *Edinburgh Medical Journal* 5 (1859-60), 967.
32. For a definition of the 'professional protection' society type see Appendix 1 - notes.
33. See *EMJ* 5 (1859-60), 967 *passim*, and 6 (1860-61), 775.
34. See Chapter Five, pp. 79–82, for more on the relationship between local societies and regional branches of the BMA.
35. These figures exclude the student medical societies, the longest lived of which is the Royal Medical Society (1737). For the duration of other student societies see Appendix 2.
36. For a further discussion on the role of the Edinburgh Obstetrical Society see Chapter Two, pp. 40–5.
37. Guthrie 'Edinburgh Pathological Club' (1966), 88.
38. Loudon and Stevens, 'Primary Care and the Hospital' ch. in John Fry (1980), 147; see also Stevens (1966), *passim.*
39. See *EMJ* 1 (1911), pp. 3-4, and also *Glasgow Medical Journal* 74 (July–December 1910), 445.
40. See programme of the Scottish Society for Experimental Medicine Golden Jubilee Meeting, 28 October 1988, pp. 24-5.
41. Constitution of the Scottish Thoracic Society (formerly Tuberculosis Society), 18 March 1921, 2, Royal College of Physicians of Edinburgh.
42. The first such 'professional protection' society identified was the short-lived Association of Scottish of Medical Practitioners (1859-61), which was discussed earlier in this Chapter.
43. Dow and Calman (1990), 102-3.
44. *GMJ* 78 (July–December, 1912), 100.
45. *Ibid.*, 80 (July–December, 1913), 120.
46. *Ibid.*, 110 (July–December, 1928), pp. 168-9.

CHAPTER TWO

The Range, Nature and Educational Aspects of Medical Society Discussion and Activity

A diverse range of medical topics was discussed in the great variety of medical societies and associations which existed at one time or another in the period between 1731 and 1939. Following the procedure of the previous Chapter which outlined seven types of medical society, this Chapter is an attempt to categorise and provide an overall structure to the wide range of medical interests touched on by a selection of societies.

The twenty-six societies chosen as exemplars for this chapter are necessarily those for which there is a good deal of surviving documentation. The societies used as the basis for analysis in this Chapter reflect the diversity of medical societies in Scotland. The division of societies by type does not imply that for instance 'single discipline' societies had much less variety in paper content. The Edinburgh Obstetrical and Glasgow Obstetrical and Gynaecological Societies for example, naturally devoted most of their time to matters relating to these branches of medicine. Yet within this area of medicine, discussions ranged from individual case histories to obituaries of departed members; from diseases of childbirth to state legislation respecting midwives; from anatomical presentations to the demonstration of new or modified instruments and drugs; and from the description of surgical operations to historical contributions on the progress of the speciality through the ages. Similar wide-ranging patterns of debate can be drawn for other apparently single–discipline and specialist societies.

CATEGORIES OF SUBJECTS DISCUSSED IN MEDICAL SOCIETIES

The most cursory perusal of the minute books and secondary publications of a single medical society reveals a great variety in the type and nature of discussions even within the space of one year, let alone in the passage of in some cases, more than two centuries. With the better administered societies there is also the problem of the great quantity of the minutes and other papers generated over a considerable length of time. How much more difficult then the task of quantifying and assessing the contents of prepared papers, verbal communications, and clinical and pathological demonstrations of the 160[1] societies which existed within the period 1731–1939. To overcome these difficulties a series of twenty-five categories was devised in which to place the various types of communications delivered to a cross-section of Scottish medical societies, and to examine how such contributions altered during the society's history.

At least one of the twenty-five categories came up at almost every meeting (other than specific extraordinary meetings), that listed as number 24 'internal affairs'. This heading refers to anything relating to the administration of the society, (including among other things; arrangements for future meetings; admission of new members; changes in constitution; alterations to membership costs; purchase of new books; and, plans for social events, e.g. annual dinners). Such concerns proved to be almost the sole, and certainly the main business of some society meetings.

Of all the categories of medical society discussion constructed, the most obvious was that of 'case history' description. The recounting of an interesting case or series of cases to a group of fellow practitioners is possibly the earliest form of mutual medical education practised outside apprenticeship or the bounds of university teaching. Such an exchange of day-to-day case work need not have taken place within the confines of a medical society, although during the eighteenth century and thereafter this was increasingly the favoured method, as case studies constituted a staple element in the growing numbers of medical societies established in Scotland. This will be demonstrated later in an examination of the contents of the transactions of some of the medical and related scientific societies. The use of transactions as a means of identifying a society's activities is not without its difficulties however, since an element of 'filtering' society discussion and debate for wider consumption through the careful selection of papers has to be considered.

> it is well known, that good papers confer honour on their authors, while, of those which are indifferent, a portion of the discredit is shared by the Society. The dignity of the scientific institution, therefore, as well as the interest of the profession and the public whom they propose to benefit, requires that they should exercise a discretionary power somewhat unlimited...[2]

One other point to be made in this brief review of the categories employed is the number of these which fall broadly under the definition 'educational'. This side to medical societies (in a variety of changing forms), remained dominant for almost the whole period, only latterly challenged by the development of institutionalised post-graduate medical education after 1914. Only three categories did not fulfil at least in part, an educational purpose for society members, one of which, 'internal' matters, has already been mentioned. The other broadly 'non-educational' categories, covering 'professional' concerns and 'medico-political' issues respectively, will be referred to periodically.

Categories of Medical Society Discussion

1. Case histories: (a) clinical; (b) surgical; (c) pathological (inc. specimens); (d) obstetrical

2. Disease: description; treatment; control

3. Obstetrical/gynaecological

4. Surgical

5. Professional/ethical

6. Medico-political

7. (a) Clinical; (b) pathological

8. Scientific/research-based

9. (a) Anatomical; (b) physiological

10. (a) Overseas work experience; (b) untitled presidential address

11. Topics of general medical or medical-related interest

12. Public health/preventive medicine/sanitation

13. Unable to categorise

14. Psychological/mental illness

15. Historical/life of a celebrated figure

16. Therapeutics: specific medicines, treatments, instruments

17. War: medical experiences, related diseases/injuries

18. Hospital reports

19. Hospital demonstrations

20. (a) Non-medical related; (b) obituaries of members

21. Demonstration of medical/scientific equipment

22. Addresses by distinguished medical guests

23. Discussions on transactions and other publications

24. 'Internal affairs': increase in membership/fees, library holdings, meeting place, social event arrangements, etc.

25. Short presentations: (a) 'foreign bodies removed'; (b) casts and drawings

VARIETY OF MEDICAL SOCIETY ACTIVITY AND DISCUSSION

The objects of the Society shall be – To receive and discuss communications on Medicine, Surgery and the allied sciences, the nature of which shall have been previously intimated to the Members by Billet; to receive, without discussion communications in regard to pathological specimens exhibited on the table, and to promote professional improvement by any other means that may, from time to time, be approved by the Society.[3]

(*Revised Laws of the Edinburgh Medico-Chirurgical Society*, 1869)

Figure 2.1: Extract from the printed Annual Report on the Forfarshire Medical Association, 3 May 1898.

CASES SHOWN—

(1) A Case after Pyaemic Arthritis.
(2) A Case after Fracture of Humeral Neck.
(3) A Case of Congenital Subluxation and Coloboma of the Lens.
(4) A Case of Dermatitis due to Pregnancy.
(5) A Case of Obscure Skin Disease.
(6) A Case of Reproduction of the Humerus after Acute Necrosis.
(7) A Case after Eslander's Operation.
(8) A Case of Congenital Malformation of the Anus rectified by Operation.
(9) A Case of Recovery after Operation for Volvulus.
(10) A Case of Incurable Malignant Tumour in Abdomen after Coeliotomy.
(11) A Case after Operation for Appendicitis with Retrocaecal Abscess.
(12) A Case after Coeliotomy for Abdominal Pain.
(13) A Case of Congenital Diplegia.

SPECIMENS SHOWN—

(1) Malignant Tumour compressing Superior Vena Cava and Right Bronchus.
(2) Tuberculous Bursae.
(3) Fibromyoma of the Ovary.
(4) Bronchoceles.
(5) Tuberculous Spleen, Liver, and Lung.
(6) Atheroma of Aorta.
(7) Careinoma of Œsophagus, Stomach, and Liver.
(8) Compressed Foetus.
(9) Haemotoma from Neck.
(10) Congenital Dislocation of the Humerus.
(11) Case of Osteoarthritis of Wrist and Ankle from a lad of thirteen.
(12) Heart showing Clots in the Superior Vena Cava and Left Subclavian Vein.
(13) Heart showing Mitral Stenosis with a Large Left Auricle
(14) An Old Standing Intra-Capsular Fracture of the Neck of the Femur.
(15) Uterus Removed by Vaginal Hysterectomy for Cancer of the Cervix.
(16) Heart with Calcification in Wall of Left Ventricle.
(17) A Series of Specimens Treated by Tore's Method.
(18) A Self-Retaining Operating Vaginal Speculum.

PAPERS READ—

(1) The Action of Piperazin on Vesical Calculi, by Dr DICKSON.
(2) A Case of Chylous Transudation into the Thoracic and Abdominal Cavities,* by Dr MACKIE WHYTE.
(3) The Disinfection of Rooms by Spraying, by Dr TEMPLEMAN.
(4) A Case of Hemiplegia, with Atrophy of the Affected Side, by Dr STALKER.
(5) Some Simple Manoeuvres for General Gynecological Practice,† by Dr BUIST.
(6) A Case of Colectomy for Obstruction,‡ by Dr MacEWAN.
(7) A Case of Asphasia following a Traumatism, by Dr MacVICAR.
(8) A Paper on Nasal Obstruction, by Dr GUILD.
(9) A Case of Labour, complicated by Ovarian Tumour, with subsequent removal by Operation, by Dr KYNOCH.
(10) A Case of Congenital Diplegia, by Dr MACKIE WHYTE.
(11) A Case of Spinal Myelitis, by Dr STALKER.
(12) A Case of Bradycardia,¶ by Dr TENNANT BRUCE.
(13) A Case of Enterectomy, with end to end Anastomosis, by Mr GREIG.
(14) A Case of Intra-Abdominal Strangulation successfully treated by Coeliotomy, by Mr GREIG.
(15) A Case of recovery from Favus, with Photo, by Mr GREIG.
(16) The Treatment of Cystocele, by Dr BUIST.
(17) A Case of Acute General Erythema following a Septic Ulcer, by Dr HALLET.
(18) A Case of Hepatic Abscess, by the RESIDENT.
(19) A Simple Method of Clinical Bacteriology,§ by Dr PIRI.
(20) A Case of Injury to the Lumbosacral Cord, by Dr FOGGIE.

Vide 'Edinburgh Medical Journal' for December 1897.
†*Vide* 'Scottish Medical and Surgical Journal' for December 1897.
‡*Ibidem* Vol. II. No. 1.   ¶*Ibidem* Vol. II. No. 4   §*Ibidem* Vol. II No. 5.

Reproduced by kind permission of the Archivist, University of Dundee.

The Discussion of Case Histories

Since the description of case work, of whatever type, looms large in the content of medical society discussion it is useful to examine the proceedings of the earliest Scottish medical society to measure how far case histories provided the staple diet of such discussion in the 1730s. The Medical Society of Edinburgh was established with the intention of improving medical knowledge through a series of published transactions made up of papers which had been heard by or communicated to, the society. In the five volumes of *Medical Essays and Observations* published between 1733 and 1744, 217 papers were included. Of these 88 (41 per cent) were case histories. Two examples from volume two of the *Medical Essays* will give a flavour of type of instructive case history included by the *Essays* editors; '"Uncommon Haemorrhagies (sic) for Twenty Nine Years", by Mr Patrick Murray, Surgeon at Earlston', and '"An Asthma, accompanied with Palpitations and flying Pains of the Breast and Shoulder", by Robert Lowis, Fellow of the College of Physicians at Edinburgh'.[4]

The Philosophical Society (of Edinburgh) despite its name and avowed original intentions to improve the level of knowledge in both arts and science, remained predominantly a medical society throughout its existence (1737–83), not unlike its immediate predecessor the Edinburgh Medical Society. The majority of papers in the Philosophical Society's three volumes of printed transactions: *Essays and Observations, Physical and Literary*; were clinical observations (including a small number on individual cases) and research based medical reports e.g. 'A description of the American Yellow Fever, in a letter from John Lining, Physician at Charles-Town, to Robert Whytt Professor of Medicine in the University of Edinburgh'[5] and 'Answer to an Objection against Inoculation [sic]; by Ebenezeer Gilchrist, Physician at Dumfries'.[6] There were also a large number of papers on anatomical and obstetrical subjects, most written by Alexander Monro *Primus* and *Secundus*.[7] As to be expected given the wider remit of the Philosophical Society, there were a small number of papers (3 per cent) on non-medical themes and a good proportion of papers, (17 per cent) on medical-related scientific subjects.

Almost a century later the early meetings of the Medical Society's later counterpart, the Edinburgh Medico-Chirurgical Society, reveal the continued importance of the discussion of bread-and-butter case work in medical societies. Of the 84 papers included in the first three volumes of its *Transactions* published between 1824 and 1829, 22 (26 per cent) were based on case histories, 12 of which were clinical and pathological, 7 obstetrical and 2 surgical. However, other types of paper received equal attention, e.g. there were 22 papers devoted to disease description and treatment: reflecting perhaps, the changing role of the general practitioner in an expanding city where the growing population would provide many cases (and on occasion epidemics) of the same disease seen by any one practitioner, whose contributions to medical society debate would similarly broaden with experience.

In the last decades of the nineteenth century (in the years 1881–5) case histories still accounted for nearly 60 per cent of the printed transactions of the

Edinburgh Medico-Chirurgical Society. Seventy-one per cent of all the case histories delivered in these years were based on the display of pathological specimens, and although showing specimens was not a new phenomenon in society activity, the proportion of time given over to this activity was considerable, representing 41 per cent of all society business reproduced in the *Transactions* of 1881–5. However, this percentage is to an extent misleading since it must be assumed that the display of a pathological specimen would take up relatively little of a meeting when compared to the reading of a paper on a given medical subject.

The preceding comments on the Edinburgh Medico-Chirurgical Society are chiefly based on evidence taken from the printed proceedings of the Society, and such printed records were not necessarily intended to be comprehensive records of society activity. Also less than 15 per cent of Scottish medical societies published transactions (the link between medical societies and collective further education notwithstanding). For example, the Aberdeen Medico-Chirurgical Society has not at any time in its 203-year history published transactions of its business. Reports of meetings were from time to time included in contemporary medical journals, but it does not seem to have been a priority for the Society to attempt to widen the audience for its intellectual debates, for reasons which are not clear. Indeed, there is very little reference to this issue contained within the Society minute books, the following passage which appeared in 1927 demonstrates the Society's apparent attitude towards the cost of regular reports of its business:

> A letter was read from the Editor of the *Edinburgh Medical Journal* submitting a scheme for the publication of the Society's transactions in that journal. It was unanimously agreed that the scheme did not come within the financial scope of the society.[8]

Fee-fixing and Professional Self-regulation

An area where the Aberdeen Medico-Chirurgical Society displayed consistent concern for having its activities more widely recorded was in the area of medical fees, tables of which were printed and made available to customers at local dispensing chemists at regular intervals. The same tables were inserted in the local press. The first such fee schedule appeared in 1816, and was renewed frequently, the minute books referring to new tables in 1829, 1842, 1846, 1849, 1863, and finally in 1916.[9] In 1818, the Medical Society of the North printed a detailed schedule of fees, with four different scales dependent upon patients social class.[10] Preoccupation with local fee levels in the course of the nineteenth century was not limited to north of Scotland practitioners. In central Scotland the Mentieth Medical Society established in 1861, listed the drawing up of a schedule of fees as one of its aims on formation.[11] In Edinburgh, the Lothians Medical Association was set up with the intention to increase the status of the profession, and one of the main ways this was to be achieved was through the regulation of fees in the locality, as an extract from the Association's constitution reprinted in the *EMJ* in April 1867 revealed:

> The general objects of the Association shall be to procure combination of

action in all matters affecting the interests of the profession... [including] recommending, and as far as may be introducing into the usage of medical men such practices in regard to fees and other matters as may best secure the interest of the members and the dignity of the profession.[12]

Just over a year later the Association published a guide to fee levels for its members. It covered ordinary visits, midwifery fees, charges for vaccinations and providing medical certificates, and the fees to be charged for the attendance of two or more patients in one house.[13] The main section of the report dealt with the various levels of fees to be imposed based on patients' income.

> the following classification of patients and rate of fees is proposed:- 'Class 1, when the house rental is under £50 per annum; class 2, from £50 to £100; class 3, from £100 upwards. That for ordinary visits and advice at practitioner's house the fees should be: class 1, 2s. 6d. to 5s.; class 2, 3s. 6d. to 7s. 6d.; class 3, 5s. to 10s. and upwards. A few visits should always be charged at the higher rates, but when the attendance is prolonged the lower rates may be taken...'[14]

Many nineteenth-century medical societies were concerned with determining a scale of fees, and there is evidence of communication between societies around the country before fixing local rates. In 1864, the Buchan Medical Society issued a table of fees[15] which had been compiled after reference to the fee levels charged by other medical societies, including the Aberdeen Medico-Chirurgical and Glasgow Medical Societies, and the Banff, Moray and Nairn, Deeside, and Garioch and Northern Medical Associations in 1863/4. A comparison of printed fee tables from all but one of the societies noted above (there is no fee table from the Glasgow Medical Society), among the records of the Buchan Medical Society shows a strong similarity in recommended minimum fees. The Buchan Medical Society, as in the four other societies (and the Lothians Medical Association in 1868), charged a minimum fee of two shillings and sixpence for a single local daytime visit. The same sum was the minimum recommended fee in all five societies for a minor surgical operation (which included tooth extraction and vaccination). A minimum one guinea fee was charged in all societies for the issue of a lunacy certificate, and in all societies apart from the Buchan, one guinea was also the minimum recommended fee (rising to a maximum of three guineas) charged for a consultation. The consultation fee in the Buchan Medical Society was much lower, at five shillings, rising to a maximum of one guinea. The area where there was most diversification was in the fee for midwifery services. The Garioch and Northern and the Banff, Moray and Nairn Medical Associations both recommended a minimum one guinea fee for non-complicated deliveries, while the Deeside Medical Association suggested twelve shillings and sixpence for an ordinary delivery. The Buchan's recommended minimum delivery fee was ten shillings and sixpence, while the Aberdeen Medico-Chirurgical Society set the lowest fee for basic midwifery provision at ten shillings. The lower level charged by the Aberdeen Society may have been due to the fact that midwifery services of varying kinds were more readily available in a large city than in some

Figure 2.2: Medical society fee tables from the 1860s.

FEE TABLE OF THE GARIOCH AND NORTHERN MEDICAL ASSOCIATION, 1863.

Single or Express Visit) – Within a mile of practitioner's residence – 2/6–5 shillings.

Ditto) – At greater distance, an extra rate of 1 shilling per mile.

Subsequent attendance, according to its length, and the distance, and social position of the patient.

Night Visit) – A Double Fee.

Detention or Special Service) – An Extra Rate.

Midwifery) – Delivery in Ordinary Cases – £1 1 shilling.

Ditto) – Delivery in Difficult Cases – an Extra Rate.

Attendance in Protracted Recovery at Visit Rate.

These fees to be paid half-yearly at Whitsunday and Martinmas.

The following to be paid when the service is rendered:-

	£	s	d
Advice) – At Practitioner's Residence	0	2	6

Surgery) – Extraction of Teeth; Vaccination; and the Minor Operations of Surgery:

	£	s	d
At Practitioner's Residence	0	2	6
At Patient's Residence (same as Single Visit)	to 5	0	0

Other Operations) – According to Importance.

	£	s	d
Necessary assistance in Midwifery or Surgical Operations) – each assistance	1	1	0
Consultation) – In Medical or Surgical Case	1	1	0
Certificates) – Ordinary Certificate	0	5	0
Ditto) – Lunacy Certificate	1	1	0
Ditto) – Insurance Reports (chargeable to Company)			
– on policies of £300	1	1	0
– Under £300	0	10	6

By Order of the Association.
Kintore Arms Inn, Inverurie,
26th September 1863.

Reproduced with the permission of the Archivist, University of Aberdeen.

BANFF, MORAY, AND NAIRN MEDICAL ASSOCIATION TABLE OF FEES

A t a GENERAL MEETING of the BANFF, MORAY, AND NAIRN MEDICAL ASSOCIATION, held at Elgin, on the 30th day of January 1864, the following TABLE was adopted, and ordered to be printed and circulated amongst the Members, and advertised in the local Newspapers:-

VISITS

	From	To
The first Visit in Town or advice at Practitioner's Residence,	£0 2 6	£0 10 6
Subsequent Attendance, to be according to its length and the Social Position of the Patient.		
Night Visit	0 5 0	1 1 0
Visit to the Country, at any distance not exceeding Two Miles	0 5 0	and upwd.
For every additional Mile, from	0 1 6	0 5 0
Night Visits to Country to be Doubled.		

	From	To
Every hour that the Practitioner is detained, either from urgency of the case, or desire of the Patient or Friends,	£0 2 6	0 5 0

It is understood that these Fees should be paid at the time of Visit, or when the attendance terminates.

	From	To
Ordinary Fee for Consultation	£1 1 0	3 3 0

The Fee for consultation or other Medical attendance, when the Practitioner is not the one regularly employed by the Family, is expected to be paid at the time of visit.

	From	To
Ordinary Medical Certificate,	£0 2 6	0 10 6
Lunacy Certificate,	1 1 0	

SURGICAL OPERATIONS AND MIDWIFERY

	From	To
Vaccination, Extraction of Teeth, Cupping, Bleeding, and other minor Operations	£0 2 6	£0 10 6
Operation of Hydrocele, Harelip, Tapping, Excision of Small Tumours, Amputation of Toes, Fingers, &c	0 5 0	2 2 0
Reducing Fractures and Dislocations,	0 10 6	3 3 0
Capital Operations, viz: Amputation, Trepanning, Aneurism, Extirpation of Mamma, Lithotomy, Lithotrity,	2 2 0	21 0 0
Necessary Assistance at Operations,	1 1 0	2 2 0
Delivery in Ordinary Cases,	1 1 0	10 10 0
Do. in Difficult or Protracted Cases,	1 11 6	10 10 0

In all cases of Operations and Midwifery, the Fee may be paid at the time, and to be independent of future visits.

Post Mortem Examination, when required by relatives, not less than   £2 2 0 of the more rural, scattered communities served by the members of the other societies.

The fixing and indeed, collection of medical fees remained an important aspect of medical society discussion into the twentieth century. In October 1925, the Glasgow Northern Medical Society held a special meeting to discuss a minimum fee scale for the area. Reference to the fees levels fixed reveal few changes in the course of sixty years. The minimum recommended fee for a single daytime visit was three shillings and sixpence, the vaccination charge remained the same as in the 1864 fee schedules at two shillings and sixpence, while the cost of a confinement 'without chloroform' had risen to two guineas.

The fee schedules devised by medical societies were recommendations issued to inform the paying public as to the cost of consulting the medical profession, as much as to avoid the undercutting of fees by rival local medical practitioners, (always providing they were members of the local medical society). It is clear by the insertion of fee schedules in local newspapers and the printing of cards with society fee schedules to be issued at local chemist shops, that the medical profession had difficulty in obtaining payment for their work. In 1850, the Glasgow Southern Medical Society purchased a 'black book' in which Society members were asked to list patients who had not paid their fees, for the information of other members.[16] In 1908, the Glasgow Western Medical Society took to employing its own debt collector to extract outstanding debts from recalcitrant patients. Members of the Society were requested to give outstanding accounts to the appointed collector, who then charged a commission of 25 per cent on all amounts collected in instalments from patients, and 10 per cent on all debts collected as a result of writing to patients, or 'debtors' as they were referred to in the Society minutes.[17]

In areas where competition for patients was high and the levels of payment consequently low, other regulatory factors were to the fore in medical societies. The early, and to some degree, abiding aim of the Glasgow Southern was the practical exchange of medical views in a social atmosphere. The early entries in the minute books stress the almost daily exchange of views and discussions of case work among a small gathering of local practitioners at a nearby coffee house.[18] The importance attached to local cooperation and mutual exchange of information by the Glasgow Southern Medical Society rather than to the wider dissemination of its medical discussions, (it published no transactions), can arguably be said to have arisen as much out of necessity as of design. The medical profession as a whole was placed under pressure as it expanded in the mid-nineteenth century, and competition for patients and for local government appointments steadily intensified. The conflict in the mid- and later nineteenth century caused in respect of Medical Officer appointments in the north of Scotland spilled over into local medical societies.

The weight attached by the Glasgow Southern Medical Society to regulating the profession from within can be measured by its construction of a 'Code of Ethics' in 1851. This was complemented by the establishment of a committee to monitor medical ethical problems within the Society's ranks. The necessity for such a committee was clearly demonstrated during the course of that year by a dispute between several society members over an undisclosed alleged breach of etiquette which led to the resignation of one the members, James Millar, a local general practitioner. In consequence of such internal conflict the Society printed three hundred copies of the *Code of Ethics and Laws of the Society*, which were circulated to every member.[19]

Competition for patients and medical posts could also be augmented by personal antagonism, as in the case of James Young Simpson, Professor of Midwifery at the University of Edinburgh and James Miller, Professor of Surgery, in 1852. Both men had seen but gave differing diagnoses on a female patient who subsequently died. The cause of her death led to an open dispute between the two medical professors and the eventual intervention of the Aesculapian Club, to which both belonged. The Club was convened in the absence of the two men and a document was drawn up to be sent to Professors Simpson and Miller stressing the injury their argument had caused to the character of the profession, and requesting that they express regret for their actions, to the extent that they provide suitable (liquid) reparation to the Club members for the disruption they had caused.[20]

Local Public Health

Interest in heightening the status of the profession through increased cooperation over fees and cases was not the only moving influence in society activity in the nineteenth century. The Aberdeen Medico-Chirurgical Society demonstrated an early and abiding concern for, and direct involvement in, local public health matters: such as the drawing up of a handbill of preventive measures to combat an unspecified 'fever epidemic' in the city in 1818. This was then printed and circulated by the local authorities.[21] The setting up of a committee to examine and grant certificates of competence to local midwives in 1827 can be taken in the same vein.[22] So too, can the appointment of two delegates from the society to serve on a local government sanitary committee to 'suppress nuisances' (i.e. remove potential health hazards), which was set up in response to the cholera epidemic which was sweeping the country in 1848.[23] In 1908, Society pressure succeeded in forcing the Town Council to amend its operation of the 1907 Notification of Births Act,[24] and ten years later it was in the vanguard of the movement to improve maternity and infant welfare in the city, holding a special meeting to outline its proposals.[25] Perhaps most notable of all was the Society meeting in 1920 at which Matthew Hay, the city's Medical Officer for Health, first detailed plans to extend and centrally locate the city's hospital accommodation, plans which led to the construction of the Foresterhill medical complex on the outskirts of the city.[26]

In common with the Aberdeen Medico-Chirurgical Society, inadequate hospital provision in the locality proved to be an issue of major concern to the Glasgow Southern Medical Society, and again a society meeting was the occasion for the launching of a campaign to increase such provision.[27] The movement for extended hospital provision for the south side of city which ultimately led to the opening of the Glasgow Victoria Infirmary in 1890, was the beginning of a close relationship between the Society and the Infirmary. In the short term this resulted in the Society being allowed to elect annually a governor to the hospital to represent the Society's interests in its administration,[28] while in the longer term, the hospital came to provide a meeting place for the Society in the 1920s.[29] In 1841, the Greenock Medico-Chirurgical Association was approached by the Trustees of Greenock Infirmary to give their opinion on two possible expansion plans for the hospital aimed at increasing the number of beds for patients.[30] The Association deferred opinion on the building proposals until they had consulted with an architect. Two months later the Association came up with its own recommendation that the Infirmary Trustees should build a 100-bed fever hospital with ceilings of a height of no less than sixteen feet:[31] the response of the Trustees to this ambitious suggestion is not recorded in the minutes.

Changes in Society Discussions in the Course of the Nineteenth Century

The general tendencies of medical societies towards the mutual improvement of the profession, by way of the wider dissemination of papers through the medium of printed transactions; through agreed fee levels within the locality; and by taking a strong interest in the level of local public health provision have been outlined, largely using isolated examples ranging across a wide timescale. But by looking at a variety of sources useful comparisons can be made of the activities of several societies in the early and later part of the nineteenth centuries.

The existence of bound copies of the papers delivered before the Glasgow Medical Society in a 28-volume series covering the years 1814–44[32] (two further volumes have been lost) allows a direct comparison to be made with the activities of the Edinburgh Medico-Chirurgical Society during the years 1824–9 (a period covered by the latter Society's first three volumes of transactions), and with the Fife Medico-Chirurgical Society for which a partial list of papers exists for the years 1826–8.[33]

Between 1825–9 84 papers were delivered before the Edinburgh society and printed in the *Transactions*, 27 (32 per cent) of these were case histories, and 22 (26 per cent) related to a variety of diseases and methods of treatment. A similar picture emerges for the Glasgow Medical Society in the same period: 56 papers survive in bound form for these years, (one volume covering parts of 1824 and 1825 is missing), and of these 16 (29 per cent) are case histories and 12 (21 per cent) relate to disease and its treatment.

Three areas where the discussions of the Glasgow Medical Society appear more comprehensive than those of the Edinburgh Medico-Chirurgical Society in these years are their inclusion of medical education;[34] hospital reports[35] (from the Glasgow Eye Infirmary and Glasgow Royal Infirmary); and on phrenology[36] which was the subject of two papers. It is possible that such topics were also the subject of discussion in the Edinburgh Medico-Chirurgical Society during these years and were simply not considered for inclusion in the printed transactions, particularly in regard to comments on medical education and phrenology which may have been considered as areas too sensitive to be published at this time. Their inclusion in the more comprehensive bound collection of papers of the Glasgow Medical Society is, however, an indication of the great range of issues addressed in the city's leading medical society.

The comparison between the activities of the Edinburgh Medico-Chirurgical Society and the Glasgow Medical Society in the late 1820s can be augmented by reference to the activities of the Fife Medico-Chirurgical Society. Unlike the other societies in this section, the source for the Fife society, although emanating from the society itself, is not a minute book or bound volume of papers delivered, or retrospective published transactions, but a printed circular sent to all Fife medical practitioners in order to promote the society and its activities, so once again, as in the case of the Edinburgh Medico-Chirurgical Society's transactions, the problem of the filtering of information on society business for wider consumption has to be considered. The *Circular for the Medical Practitioners of Fife*, printed in Cupar in October 1828, contains a list of fourteen papers delivered before the Society between 1826 and 1828. The preamble to the list of papers delivered reveals the degree of selectivity demonstrated by the *Circular*'s compiler:

> During the short period that has elapsed since its formation the following essays have been read before the Society, *besides numerous interesting but less extended communications* [my emphasis]...[37]

Seven of the fourteen essays listed were on physiological subjects, such as 'Essay Containing some General Remarks on the Physiology of the Nervous System, by Mr Adam Wisemann, Surgeon, Cupar – January 1827'.[38] Others dealt with disease, medical topography, the life of Alexander Monro *Secundus*, and medical insurance for the working classes.[39] A final paper of some significance was that delivered by Mr Bonnar, Surgeon from Auchtermuchty, on, '... the present condition of the Medical Profession, in regard to their intercourse with each other and the Public'.[40] From this paper and those of the Glasgow Medical Society, it is clear that 'professional concerns', including those of intra-professional competition and the position of medical education, had a place in medical societies alongside concerns for the 'mutual improvement' of the local profession at a relatively early period (the 1820s) in their history.

Reference to the records of three later nineteenth century societies: the Buchan Medical Society; the Garioch and Northern Medical Association (GNMA); and the Scottish Midland and Western Medical Association (SMWMA); none of which were based in large population centres, suggest that such medico-political and professional matters were regularly brought up for discussion in the second half of the century, alongside more day-to-day medical concerns in the locality.

From the records of the Buchan Medical Society and the GNMA it would appear that surgical case histories and papers were initially dominant. The first minuted medical paper delivered at the GNMA in November 1854 was 'Resection [partial removal] of the knee joint with successful issue' by William Keith, senior surgeon at Aberdeen Royal Infirmary.[41] Meanwhile, in the Buchan Medical Society the subject for discussion at its second annual meeting in 1863 was 'Bloodletting'. The Society's secretary somewhat ambiguously recorded, 'It was universally agreed that Bloodletting was suitable in some cases [and] that in others it was entirely out of the question...'[42]

Alongside such discussions on medical matters both societies also on occasion aired questions of local medical ethics ('medical etiquette' was the phrase used in both societies' records), as society members came into conflict as they competed for public appointments. In the case of the Buchan Medical Society, the problem, involving competition for the positions of Parochial Medical Officers in Peterhead in 1864, remained confidential, and the minute book entry is, no doubt deliberately brief.[43] In the GNMA a similar problem was given a higher profile in the Society minutes stretching from September 1888 to May 1889.

> Dr Mortimer, Turiff, brought before the meeting, the case of a medical man, a member of the Association, applying for a public medical appointment [Turiff Parochial Medical Officer] held by others.[44]

The matter according to the minutes of May 1889 was settled amicably and no members felt the need to resign from the society, but the fact that such acrimonious competition existed demonstrates the role of local medical societies as adjudicators for the profession.

In the twenty-two years within the period 1873–1932 according to the SMWMA minute book,[45] 77 papers were read or discussions held. Of these 28 (36 per cent) were on medico-political matters, and seventeen (22 per cent) referred to 'professional' issues (this figure includes questions of medical ethics). Other than private society business, which accounted for a further 27 discussions (35 per cent), only three other categories of society activity were mentioned: two scientific/research based papers were presented; as was one paper on war medical experiences, in the shape of John Lithgow's (Factory Surgeon and Captain in the Territorial Royal Army Medical Corps) Presidential Address in 1919[46] on his experiences in Gallipoli and Egypt. One final paper was delivered by an invited guest, John Baxter Gaylor, a local practitioner in Hamilton, who in 1932, described the work of a hospital in Munich.[47]

The dominance of medico-political and professional concerns in the SMWMA is shown by reference to an early minute book entry which displays the twin concerns of the Association,

> On the motion of Dr Moffat (Falkirk) seconded by Mr Stewart (Greenock) a deputation, consisting of the President, Vice-Presidents, Treasurer and Secretary, were appointed to visit upon the Right Honourable Edward J. Gordon M.P. for the Universities of Glasgow and Aberdeen, to place before him the views of the Association with regard to the increase of the fees usually paid for Post Mortem Examinations & Reports; and payment of a fee for the Certificates of Death required by the Registrar of Deaths, and the removal of the penalties attached to refusal to grant the same.

> Dr Sloan introduced the important subject of the establishment of a sick

fund for invalided medical men, which was referred to the Council for their consideration.[48]

At the end of the last century, a decision by the Glasgow Southern Medical Society to hold clinical meetings and make visits to wards of local Glasgow hospitals signals what quickly became an integral part of medical societies, the 'clinical night'.[49] This aspect of society activity continued until well into the twentieth century, with visits to specialist hospitals being added to regular Infirmary meetings[50] (although this later round of visiting may also have owed something to the commercial interests of the hospitals in question since the majority of the Southern's members were general practitioners who would from time to time in the course of their practice have to refer patients to hospital). Clinical meetings held in hospitals around the city also serves as an illustration of the shifting balance between the local societies and the teaching hospitals as centres for the continuing education of medical practitioners as the twentieth century progressed.

However, not all clinical meetings of societies were held in hospitals, society minutes from earlier in the century, when meetings were often held in individual members homes, refer to patients, some with anatomical abnormalities, shown before members. For example, in 1849, a child of fourteen days born without thumbs was exhibited before the Edinburgh Medico-Chirurgical Society.[51] It is somewhat surprising to find that the private display of patients was continued at the end of the nineteenth and in the first two decades of the twentieth century. The Dundee Clinical Club set up in 1893, displayed patients, sometimes several, at its meetings, all of which took place at members' houses. At an early meeting of the Club in 1894, David Middleton Greig (Assistant Surgeon, Dundee Royal Infirmary), in addition to reading three sets of case notes, and displaying an amputated foot removed due to the effects of gangrene, '… showed a case of a forty five year old man with a growth on his neck'.[52] Such examples imply much docility on the part of working class patients, or perhaps reflect their hopes of free medical treatment.

Medical societies were not restricted to the discussion of 'interesting cases' which occurred in general practice. Their other activities included, the determination of local fee schedules, an involvement in local public health matters, particularly in hospital provision, and in some societies, the dissemination of its discussions through the publication of transactions.

THE CONVIVIAL ASPECTS OF MEDICAL SOCIETIES

The Scottish Midland and Western Medical Association was mentioned earlier in the context of its high percentage of papers on medico-political and professional matters. Yet the Association is also noteworthy in that it became primarily a dining club after 1921, as the more serious professional and political aspects of its meetings lessened and were replaced by the holding of an annual dinner. Other medical clubs were expressly formed for the purpose of intra-professional socialising. This aspect of medical cooperation and organisation is a vital part of

Figure 2.3: Taken from the programme of the annual dinner of the Octogenarian Club, Edinburgh, 1902.

CASEBOOK—OCTOGENARIAN WARD, 1902

No	Name	Age	Occupation	Complaining of	Characterised by	Diagnosis
1	R.A.	28	Gentleman	Nothing	Risus Amabilis	Contentia Vera
2	R.O A.	6039	What *able* for	The West	The Same	Nostalgia
3	F.D.B.	38	Saint	Dragons	Stars	Honoris causá
4	N.T.B.	82(?)	Eh?	Ah!	Imp'm	Oh!
5	T.B.	36	Meatman	T.B.'s	Bs Ts	D.T.
6	J.C.D.	7 days	Lag	Calories	Skilly	Propter Quod.
7	H.M.D.	30	Mother's help	Hives	Colic	Hydrarg, c Crerâ
8	S.C.F.	37	General	Jimp Neck	Low Colars	Cervicitus.
9	W.F.	33	Fruiterer	Birthdays	Redundancy	Amicus Mulieris.
10	W.F.	33	Chef	Puddings	The Past	Periproctitis.
11	G.L.C.	36	Bleeder	Bleeding	Blood	Bloody.
12	F.W.N.H.	32	Unmentionable	Narrow Brim	Tongs	Dystocia.
13	J.M.B.H.	101	Barber-Chirurgeon	Loss of Hair	Glossy Scalp	Alopecia Lucids.
14	R.H.	34	Flesher	Bodily Want	Pickling	Pics.
15	H.H.L.	16	Filial	Words	Cacoethes Loquendi	Diarrhoea Verborum
16	G.O.C.Mac	87	Scholar	Ettles	ships	PiL Ferri.
17	D.M.	3	Miner	Feet	??	Hypothyreoidism.
18	R.M.	33	Corbie	Accent	'Doon the Watter'	Glesca.
19	D.N.P.	34	Keit	Peers	Lordosis	Myelitis Nobilis.
20	H.P.	50	Pediatrics	Weight	Cwts.	Corporiety.
21	R.P.	34	Beadle	A Figure	Swellings	Adiposis Dolorosa.
		Cf. 2 Kings				
22	A.T.S.	ix 14	Jehu	Motors	Damoa	Autophobia
23	H.J.S.	33	Carver	Kids	Cuts	Evisceratio.
24	R.s.	30	Ajax	Lightning	Defiance (not affiance)	Arsenate of Lead.
25	A.L.T.	39	Piper	Polly Pye	Snares	Nil Bonum.
		Bought				
26	H.A.T.	1886	T(ripper)	Change of Air	Drums Ooch!	Tinnitus Aurium.
27	J.U.T.	31	Paranoiac	Existence	Placidity	Eupepsia.
28	R.T.	37	Cantor	Kafooralum	Relapses	Pueila Barbi.
		Past Dis-				
29	T.T.	temper	Priest	Hue	Black	Spectaculum.
30	D.W.	34	Bachelor	The Sex	Erubescence	Misogynis.
31	G.W.	89	(So called)Expert	Definition	Sorrow	Verba Noctis.
32	N.W.	34	Ass.(Brit. Med.)	Brain(g)	As in 9	Concillitis.

Reproduced by kind permission of the Archivist, Royal College of Physicians, Edinburgh.

the evolution of the profession, particularly as it evolved through the Scottish medical schools, and it is no coincidence that the first convivial medical clubs were formed in the eighteenth century in Edinburgh, a time when the medical school of the University enjoyed a high international reputation.[53]

Such medical clubs continued to play a role in maintaining professional links between graduates of the medical schools. The Octogenarian Club (1891-1939)[54] set up in Edinburgh and open only to those who had qualified in medicine during the 1880s, demonstrates the continuity of the desire to maintain professional links first established in student days. Other convivial clubs while expressing no direct bond with past student days displayed the high-jinks mentality often associated with medical student activity, as the following extracts from the minutes of the Granton Medical Club (1841–53) demonstrate:

The Fourth meeting of the Granton Medical Club was held to day, and as usual the afternoon was brilliant, both in the fineness of the weather, and the lively conduct of the members. Before dinner, several active gentlemen, chiefly the more elderly members of the Club, had a constitutional walk on Granton Pier, and the propriety of a swimming match before the dinner of next year was recommended.

During dinner, the conversation was lively, interesting and varied. All medical matters were excluded, with a slight exception in honour of the Physiology of Digestion.... an ex-President of the Royal College of Surgeons of Edinburgh... when walking near the Hotel, was hailed from a window and persuaded to enter the Club-room. The Force required to Project an unwilling President from the window was found to be beyond all previous calculation, although each member was intensely excited, with the exception of one grand physician, whose composure would have been much admired, had it not been remembered that he was just behaving as if he stood among the patients of his own asylum.[55]

Medical Clubs also had a more serious side to their activities, in helping to promote a friendly atmosphere between rival practitioners, and thus reduce possible tension within the local profession. The example, noted earlier in this chapter, of the Aesculapian Club's intervention in a professional dispute between two club members in 1852, demonstrates this serious side to convivial activity. The objects of the Dundee Medical Club, set up in 1881, serve to reinforce the regulatory aspect of medical social clubs, '[The Club was formed] ... for the lessening of that friction among members of our profession which so frequently occurs where individual interests are involved...'.[56]

Many of the medical clubs formed in the eighteenth and nineteenth centuries retained an element of exclusivity. The Granton Medical Club extended membership by invitation only,[57] and others excluded candidates whose election was not unanimously supported.[58] The possibility is that such exclusive clubs were informally used for the purposes of extending patronage for university and hospital appointments, although such politicking remains beneath the surface of their recorded minutes.

OBSTETRICS AS A FEATURE OF SPECIFIC INTEREST IN MEDICAL SOCIETY
DISCUSSIONS

The formation of the Edinburgh Obstetrical Society in 1840 was part of the campaign by interested local practitioners and lecturers on the subject to enhance the status of this branch of medicine in Scotland. A chair of Midwifery at Edinburgh University (and the consequent acceptance of obstetrics as an integral part of the medical curriculum) had been set up only ten years previously after a long campaign aimed at the Town Council who controlled University appointments at this time (see Chapter Three, p. 61), by the City Professor of Midwifery, James Hamilton. The opposition to the chair's creation had come from the medical representatives on the Senate who '... considered that the diseases of women and children were in the province of those who taught the practice of medicine'.[59] In 1840, James Young Simpson was elected to the chair of Midwifery by a majority of one.

> There were political undercurrents and it was suggested by some that the Whigs wanted Simpson to succeed only to keep him out of another appointment.... As Professor of Midwifery he was bound to encounter opposition from those who held chairs which had been established much earlier.[60]

The Obstetrical Society was set up with Simpson as its Vice President at a time when both his own individual position, and that of the discipline were by no means fully recognised by the medical elite: the desire for increased status as well as educational concerns lay behind the Society's birth. Simpson was not behind the Society's formation, but applied for membership at its first meeting in 14 January 1840, although there had previously been a number of preliminary meetings of during December 1839.

> It was on 4th December 1839 that a meeting was held in the New Town Dispensary, Thistle Street, for the purpose of considering the propriety of establishing an Obstetrical Society in Edinburgh. It seems to have been a movement originating chiefly among the younger members of the profession who were practising Midwifery, and who were dissatisfied with the position that branch of Medicine held in the eyes of the profession and of the public, and who were anxious and determined to make an effort to raise it to a position more worthy of the important interests it guarded and the onerous duties it performed.[61]

Reference to the original laws of the Society reinforce this notion of a desire for increased status:

> 1. The Object of the Edinburgh Obstetrical Society shall be to advance Obstetric Medicine by holding Meetings for the purpose of receiving communications and conversing on subjects connected with that branch of the Profession. In furtherance of this object each member is expected to communicate to the Society such interesting Cases in that Department as may fall under his notice, and to exhibit any Morbid Specimens of interest that he may meet with. All communications are understood to be strictly confidential.
>
> 2. The Society shall consist only of persons actually engaged in the Practice of Midwifery, and who possess a Medical or Surgical Diploma.[62]

During the first year of its meeting the Edinburgh Obstetrical Society covered a somewhat limited range of topics: obstetrical and clinical case histories were notably prominent. Indeed, the first paper read before the Society in January of that year was a case of 'Spontaneous change in presentation'[63] delivered by William Beilby, Assistant Physician at the Royal Dispensary in Edinburgh. Items exhibited before the Society during its first months included pathological specimens and a set of modified forceps which had found favour with one of the members. Towards the end of 1840 the subject of publishing the Society's transactions was raised:

It was moved by Dr Simpson, seconded by Mr Zeigler – that a publishing committee be chosen for the purpose of making such abstracts of the transactions of the Society *as it deemed desirable to publish* [my emphasis].[64] In fact, no proceedings were published by the society individually until a single volume in 1847. A further solitary volume of proceedings was issued in 1867, and it was not to be until 1871 that the society finally began an annual series of transactions. From 1841 however, regular reports of society business were prepared by the publication committee for inclusion in the *Edinburgh Monthly Journal of Medical Science*. The emphasised passage above gives further evidence of the importance of treating society reports and publications with circumspection, given the understandable desire of the publishing committee to include only those papers which reflected highly on the contributions of its members.

The 1847 volume of *Edinburgh Obstetrical Society Proceedings* (which was a reprint of reports included in the *Monthly Journal*) offers a more detailed list of papers and presentations before the Obstetrical Society in the previous year than can be found in the partial record provided by the Society's own minute book, for there are no minutes extant to cover the period April 1846–January 1847. The majority of papers continued to be based around individual case notes and observations although there were papers on other issues such as epidemic fever and scurvy, and a new type of vaccinating instrument. A statistical report by Simpson was also included in the *Proceedings* which described the first two years' work at the Edinburgh Maternity Hospital, first opened in St. John Street in May 1844, and subsequently removed to Milton House, Canongate in 1846.

Also included was a series of four papers, again written by Simpson (who remained President from 1842–57), on the use of ether as an anaesthetic during labour.[65] These papers published in the year that Simpson outlined his discovery of the anaesthetic properties of chloroform at a meeting of the Edinburgh Medico-Chirurgical Society,[66] are important as early examples of the contemporary discussion on the merits and preferred methods of anaesthetic treatments in surgery and the resistance to its use in midwifery, then exciting much debate and some controversy in medical circles.[67] A discussion on the best method of administering this anaesthetic was taken up by Simpson, and James Syme, Professor of Clinical Surgery at Edinburgh University, in the Edinburgh Medico-Chirurgical Society in 1850, when the latter was President. Both men agreed that the number of fatalities could be lessened, a factor which caused much contemporary opposition to the use of anaesthetics, through improved methods of administration, and by ensuring the purity of the drug.[68] Simpson continued to make reports on his pioneering use of chloroform, describing its relative merits in several papers before the Obstetrical Society.[69]

Matters of contemporary obstetrical and gynaecological interest were not solely the remit of the Obstetrical Society, for midwifery and the treatment of the diseases of women were integral parts of general practice. In fact, controversy over the operation of ovariotomy led to tense scenes in the Edinburgh Medico-Chirurgical Society in 1845. This heroic operation was opposed by many surgeons on the medical grounds that it would prove fatal due to the infection likely to arise on opening the abdomen, (this in the period before anaesthesia and antiseptic surgery were introduced), and on the moral grounds that it removed a woman's capability to have children, and therefore challenged her acknowledged position in society.

> Of all the therapeutic innovations introduced in gynaecology during the nineteenth century, ovariotomy was undoubtedly the one which met the greatest opposition from medical practitioners and the lay public. This is as might be expected, for the ovaries were the 'grand organs' of sexual activity in women, the source and symbol of femininity itself; their removal 'unsexed' women, thus threatening deeply held beliefs about woman's nature, her social role and moral responsibilities.[70]

The sharp conflict between those who favoured the operation and those opposed to its practice come into view in the obituary of Peter Handyside, who was one of the early pioneers of this operation in Edinburgh while surgeon at the Royal Infirmary.

> He operated first in 1845, in private, in a well-known case, to which he was called by Dr. Bennett when the other surgeons had declined to operate, and with success so far as the operation was concerned [the woman died on the 70th post-operative day], although it was done by the large incision. Professors Simpson and Goodsir, Drs Campbell, Bennett, and others, were present at the operation. It may serve to show the complete change which has taken place in professional opinion in regard to the propriety of this operation, to mention, that we recollect that when Dr. Handyside read an account of this case at the Edinburgh Medico-Chirurgical Society, the other surgeons, to mark their disapproval of the operation, left the room when Dr. Handyside rose to read his paper.[71]

The case notes were reported in full in the *Edinburgh Medical Surgical Journal* the following year.[72] Both John Hughes Bennett (at that time lecturer on pathology and the practice of physic, later Professor of the Institutes of Medicine and Clinical Medicine at Edinburgh University) who was in charge of the case and Handyside, who operated, defended the operation of ovariotomy in this case, despite the unsuccessful outcome for the patient, Bennett commenting, '... I am still of the opinion that ovariotomy is warrantable *when the diagnosis of the tumour is certain and other circumstances favourable* [author's italics]'.[73] Handyside concluded the case notes by adding, 'Lastly, I must protest against the indiscriminate performance of the operation, and in such rare cases as the present, *but in such only* [author's italics], I am quite ready to repeat it'.[74] Handyside made no reference to the extreme reaction of some members of the Edinburgh Medico-Chirurgical Society when he and Bennett read their report on the case, in his presidential valedictory address before the Society in 1874, which was in the shape of a review of the Society's history since 1821, although he did refer to the paper itself.[75]

The changing interests of the Edinburgh Obstetrical Society in the course of the nineteenth century may be measured by reference to a volume of *Transactions* (volume 21, 1896), published almost exactly fifty years after the first *Proceedings* reached the press in 1847. Communications included in this volume were divided into separate sections for obstetrics and gynaecology, although at least one paper was wrongly cited in both: 'Experimental Research into the action of *Viburnum Prunifolium* (Black Haw), [a bark extract used to treat painful menstruation]',[76] which was delivered before the society by Theodore Shennan (a recently graduated practitioner, formerly non-Resident Clinical Clerk at Edinburgh Royal Infirmary). Individual cases continued to be presented in both obstetrics and gynaecology and there were two papers on modified midwifery forceps.[77] Another paper of some interest, and one presumably communicated rather than read to the Society, came from Surgeon-Captain C. H. Bedford, of the Indian Medical Service, Bombay, which dealt with 'Criminal Abortion in the Punjab',[78] which serves as an example of the international scope of Scottish medical society interest and discussion.

Most prominence in the volume was given to a major enquiry in three parts into Teratogenesis (the production of physical defects in the foetus) and the causes of monstrosities by John William Ballantyne (Secretary of the Obstetrical Society, and lecturer on Midwifery and Diseases of Women, Medical College for Women, Edinburgh), who also happened to be Editor of the *Transactions* for the year. Interest in monstrous births was nothing new for the medical profession, or indeed the general public:

> Popular and learned interest in monsters did not originate in the early modern period. There was a long tradition of writing on the subject, both in classical and Christian antiquity and during the Middle Ages.... By the end of the 17th century, monsters had lost their links with earthquakes and the like, and had been integrated into the medical disciplines of comparative anatomy and embryology.[79]

The study of monsters had a long history in Scottish medical debate also, as shown in the volume of *Essays and Observations, Physical and Literary* of the Philosophical Society for 1756: included among the papers was, 'The Description of a monstrous Foetus; by John Mowat, Surgeon at Langholm, in a letter to Alex. Monro senior, M.D. and P.A.',[80] which began:

> Several learned men having of late years disputed about the formation of monsters, it is probable the histories of them may be of use in accounting for some phenomena in nature; on this account I send you the following description of one...[81]

Mowat's depiction of a set of female Siamese twins joined at the navel was of sufficient interest to attract Monro *secundus* who was at this time sharing the chair of Anatomy at Edinburgh University with his father, to conduct an anatomical examination of the foetus which had been preserved and a wax model made of its figure.[82]

If obstetrical matters had been, and continued to be, subjects for discussion for the wider medical population, the Obstetrical Society too, debated matters of wider importance for medicine: as in 1863 when a smallpox epidemic in Edinburgh led the Society to successfully call on the Town Council for the implementation of Vaccination legislation.[83] In 1867, James Young Simpson delivered an address on the 'Construction and Salubrity of Maternity Hospitals' before the Society, in which he suggested that a new maternity hospital was needed for the city, and that it should be built on the 'cottage hospital' system, with each room limited to three beds, with a ratio of one nurse for every two or three patients. He also suggested that special provision ought to be made for the immediate removal and isolation of cases of puerperal fever as they arose.[84] These ambitious proposals echo the activities of other societies in pressing for increased local hospital provision. Although Simpson's scheme was not implemented, it demonstrated an abiding concern within the Society to improve the standard of hospital provision for midwifery cases in the city, and to lessen the threat of puerperal fever in childbirth, the danger of which remained a constant concern for midwifery cases until the introduction of sulphonamides in 1935. In 1881, the Society held a general discussion on the appliance of the principles of 'Listerism' to obstetrical practice, at a time when the benefits of antiseptic conditions were not universally accepted.[85] Lister's principals were supported in a paper by John Halliday Croom, (Physician at Edinburgh Royal Maternity Hospital, and Lecturer on Midwifery and the Diseases of Women at Edinburgh Medical School) entitled 'the Systematic Use of Antiseptics in Midwifery'.[86]

An examination of a selection of papers given before the Glasgow Obstetrical and Gynaecological Society within the period 1886-1930 suggests that this Society shared in large measure the preoccupations of its Edinburgh counterpart. Evidence to support this conclusion may be drawn from the very full listing of papers given in *The Official Year-Book of Scientific and Learned Societies of Great Britain and Ireland* for 1901. Of 44 papers cited for this year, 21 were case histories. A paper of special interest among those given on various other medical topics was an address delivered before the Society by David Yellowlees (Physician Superintendent at Glasgow Royal Asylum, Gartnavel, and lecturer on Insanity at Glasgow University) on 'Insanity and its relation to obstetrics and gynaecology'.[87] This is an early example of an address by a distinguished medical practitioner by special invitation of a medical society, something which became a notable feature of society meetings as the twentieth century progressed. Such addresses were aimed as much at enhancing the prestige as of a society as at providing as wide a range of educational opportunities as possible for their members.

While addresses by distinguished medical guests were a relatively new phenomenon at this time, there was also a great deal of continuity in society debates. In the 1920s, the Glasgow Obstetrical and Gynaecological Society displayed a remarkable degree of continuity with earlier nineteenth concerns in this field of medicine; eg. 'Labour in the case of a Thoracophagus Monster',[88] by Robert Aim Lennie (Assistant Visiting Obstetrician, Glasgow Royal Maternity and Women's Hospital); and 'Puerperal Infection in Maternity Hospitals',[89] by

Alexander McGregor OBE (Medical Officer for Health, Glasgow), would not have seemed out of place in nineteenth century society discussions, (although the contents of such papers would no doubt have been different). On the other hand, contemporary issues and treatments were also being fully discussed by the Society at this time. In 1925, the Society had a wide-ranging discussion, spread over two meetings, on '... the Future of Domestic Midwifery Practice, with special reference to a State Medical Service'.[90] New medical treatments too found their way (as they had always done) into the discussions of the Society, e.g., 'The Treatment of Cancer of the Uterus with Radium',[91] by George Thomson Mowat (Assistant Surgeon, Royal Cancer Hospital, Glasgow) and Alexander Arthur Charteris (Donald Research Scholar for Cancer, Pathology Department, Glasgow Royal Infirmary).

Throughout the 1920s individual case histories continued to be presented to the Society, and in this area the fact that there is no great move away from this earliest form of medical society communication underlines the continued role of general practitioners in every-day obstetrical practice. This is not to suggest that specialists did not play an increasingly material role in the proceedings of the society, but to imply that the continuing inclusion of individual case presentations ensured that general practitioner members of the Society could remain active participants, rather than merely onlookers waiting to be enlightened by their more eminent colleagues.

A parallel may be drawn at this point with the Royal Medico-Chirurgical Society of Glasgow, which late in the 1930s also displayed a continued concern for the interests and involvement of general practitioners. The printed Society notice for the session running from October 1937 to May 1938, includes among a list of forthcoming meetings, not only special clinical, pathological and hospital 'nights', but also two 'General Practitioner's Nights': the first was a 'Demonstration of Cardio-Vascular Diseases' held at the Southern General Hospital on 3 December 1937 with 55 cases on view in the wards; and the second, held on 4 March 1938, was a lecture on 'Some Observations on Ante-Natal Care'[92] delivered by Robert Lennie, mentioned above as a contributor to the *Transactions* of the Glasgow Obstetrical and Gynaecological Society in 1926, by this time Chief Obstetrical Surgeon at Glasgow Royal Maternity Hospital.

The discussion of obstetrics in medical societies has been highlighted to illustrate how a specific area of interest was covered in medical societies. The approach was largely one of general interest in the field. Not surprisingly, 'Scottish specialist' societies formed in the early twentieth century were more technical in their approach to particular branches of medicine.

MEDICAL SCIENCE AND MEDICO-SCIENTIFIC SOCIETIES

Mention was made earlier of the use of anaesthesia in the practice of surgery and midwifery. In a similar vein, the increased use of the microscope by medical practitioners in the 1880s can be seen in meetings held in the Edinburgh Medico-Chirurgical Society and reported in the collected transactions of the period. Further evidence for the growth in personal scientific research by general practitioners may be taken from the establishment of two microscopical societies in Scotland around this time: the Microscopical Society of Glasgow in 1886, and the Edinburgh-based Scottish Microscopical Society in 1891. While these societies contained non-medical members and sometimes included presentations of limited medical interest, e.g. 'The Metamorphosis of Insects',[93] by John Rankin (a local practitioner in Glasgow), and those of no apparent medical interest or application, e.g. 'The Microscopic Evidences of a Dry Climate in British Plants' by G. T. S. Ellis MA, FLS.,[94] other papers delivered were of significance for their medical members; 'Changes in the Ovum, preparatory to Fertilisation'[95] by Thomas H. Bryce (Lecturer on Anatomy to Women, Glasgow University), and, 'The Inter-Communicable Diseases common to Man and the Lower Animals'[96] by John Glaister, (Regius Professor of Forensic Medicine and Public Health, Glasgow University).

Less than one-third of the papers given at the Scottish Microscopical Society over the twenty year period between 1893 and 1913 had no apparent medical interest.[97] The other two-thirds covered medical topics ranging from anatomical investigations and pathological presentations to a discourse on 'The Rise of Histology in Italy'[98] by David Fraser-Harris (Council member of the Society, and Lecturer in Physiology and Histology at St. Andrews University). Other medical or medical-related papers dealt with new or advanced techniques in microscopy, although most papers read were 'scientific' or 'research-based'.[99]

The eventual decline in the number of medical presentations towards the end of this twenty year period was matched by a decline in the Society's overall vigour. From a high point of 21 papers listed as delivered in one year (1896) in the *Year-Book*, only four of which were non-medical, the society apparently reached its lowest ebb in 1910 when only five papers were read, none of which were directly medical. Also, in 1910, the hitherto annual *Proceedings* of the society became a bi-annual publication. The Society ended in 1921, with no meetings having being held during 1914–18 on account of the war. The declining involvement of the medical profession in these societies may have been due to a combination of causes, including the rise of the professional pathologist working in hospital laboratories; the increased use of microscopic research in hospital-based medical teaching; and the spread of microscopic investigation in ordinary training; factors which would render much of the investigative work undertaken by enthusiastic general practitioners obsolete in terms of medico-scientific research.

LINKS WITH THE INTERNATIONAL MEDICAL WORLD

The link between Scottish medical societies and the international medical world can be traced from the Medical Society of Edinburgh which had its published proceedings translated into French and Dutch and which included a section on 'Societies lately formed for the Improvement of Physick' citing the establishment of medical societies in France, Sweden, Germany and Hungary in its first volume.[100] The Philosophical Society's *Essays and Observations* published between 1754 and 1771 also contained four papers communicated from the American Colonies and the West Indies, presumably written by former Edinburgh medical school students, since they were sent in the form of letters to the Professors of Anatomy: Monro *primus*; and of Medicine: Robert Whytt.[101]

The notion of creating and maintaining links with the profession overseas, (and indeed, elsewhere in Great Britain and Ireland) remained strong in Scottish medical societies into the nineteenth century. The Laws of the Edinburgh Obstetrical Society indicate how clearly this need was felt, particularly in a medical discipline seeking recognition.

> With the view of securing the co-operation of individuals distinguished in medicine, who reside at a distance, the Society may confer on such persons the honorary title of 'Corresponding Members'.[102]

The list of corresponding fellows of the Society for the 1895–6 session of the Society, reveals that of 81 such members 40 were overseas members hailing from (or more commonly, working in) areas as distant as Cairo, St. Petersburg, Bombay, China, Montreal, Australia, and the Cape of Good Hope.[103]

Of course, it would be wrong to imagine that such overtures to the international medical community were all one way traffic. James Young Simpson became a corresponding member of the Medical Society of Ghent in 1836,[104] was elected an honorary member of the Berlin Obstetrical Society in 1847,[105] and in 1853 was elected a Foreign Associate of the prestigious Academie de Medicine de Paris.[106] Although Simpson is not a typical example it was not unusual for practitioners to apply for membership of overseas medical societies, particularly since personal visits to overseas Universities in the course of their study was not uncommon.

It was suggested earlier that many of the corresponding members of Scottish medical societies were Scots or Scottish-qualified, practitioners working overseas. The early volumes of the Edinburgh Medico-Chirurgical Society's *Transactions* provide a complete list of members for the year. In the year 1829 the society had 103 ordinary members and 139 corresponding members: 43 of whom were Scots-based; 45 lived in England; and 3 in Ireland. Of the remaining 48 members: 16 were from European countries (most of whom were European medical practitioners, judging by their surnames), and 9 practised in the West Indies, with only one correspondent from Northern America. Another substantial group of overseas members were the 9 Army and 3 Navy surgeons. Their contributions to the *Transactions* included: 'Diseases of the British Troops during the Burma War', by Assistant-Surgeon Walsh of the 89th Regiment, and; 'Hospital Gangrene [arising from the Peninsula War]', by J. Boggie M.D., Surgeon to the Forces'.[107] By 1882 the membership lists of the Society had become more clearly defined: there were 161 ordinary members; 168 non-resident members; 19 United Kingdom corresponding members; 42 Foreign corresponding members (most of whom were European; and 9 honorary members (a distinction granted only to figures of international standing in medicine from Britain or elsewhere).

International links were continued into the twentieth century in the activities of Scottish medical societies often with members recounting experiences of overseas work or study visits, or in the shape of visiting medical practitioners speaking as invited guests at society meetings. Links with the international medical world were also augmented by attendance at overseas medical conferences either as interested individuals reporting their experience, or as official representatives of Scottish societies: selection for such travel was no doubt regarded as an honour.

> It was agreed [by the Council of the Edinburgh Medico-Chirurgical Society] that Dr. Affleck [Consultant Physician at Edinburgh Royal Infirmary and the City Hospital] is to be recommended to be the Society's delegate at the forthcoming International Medical Congress in Berlin.[108]

As the twentieth century progressed and methods of communication and travel improved, links between Scottish societies and the international medical community strengthened. The Medical Women's Federation which was established in 1917, and which included two (later three) local Scottish associations,[109] was in 1919 a founder member of the Medical Women's International Federation.[110] The Scottish connection was to the forefront when the Medical Women's International Association, as the organisation had become known by this time, held its fourth annual congress at the Royal College of Physicians in Edinburgh in July 1937 with delegates from 23 countries in attendance.[111]

Most of this chapter has emphasised the broadly 'educational' nature of medical society discussion, presentation and proceedings. However, medical societies had many other concerns, including the defence of professional interests, exerting political pressure, fixing fees, and the organisation of social events. Similarly it is clear that medical societies, although contained broadly within the confines of the process of mutual and continuing education (the former chiefly in the eighteenth and nineteenth centuries, and the latter in the twentieth), covered a great variety of subjects allied to the practice of medicine as it developed over a period of 200 years, and in reflecting the diversity and range of areas with which the medical profession was concerned, medical societies provide a vital insight into its development.

NOTES

1. See Appendices 1 and 2 for a chronological list of the senior and student and graduate medical societies in this survey. See also Part Two for individual entries for the societies.
2. Review of first volume of the *Transactions of the Edinburgh Medico-Chirurgical Society EMSJ* 21 (1824), 218.
3. Revised Laws of the Edinburgh Medico-Chirurgical Society (Edinburgh, 1869), Edinburgh University Library, Special Collections Department.
4. *Medical Essays* Vol. 2 (1752), pp. vi, vii.
5. See *Essays and Observations* Vol. 2 (1756), pp. 370-95.
6. *Ibid.*, pp. 396-402.
7. There were thirteen papers on anatomical and obstetrical subjects, in the *Essays and Observations*, nine of which were written by the two Monros. See *Essays and Observations*, Vols 1-3 (1754, 1756, 1771) *passim*.

8. Aberdeen Medico–Chirurgical Society minute book, 2 June 1927, Manuscript Collection, Aberdeen University Library.
9. Aberdeen Medico–Chirurgical Society *op.cit.*, minute book, 19 December 1816, and *passim.*
10. Rules adopted by the Medical Society of the North (Inverness, 1818).
11. *Stirling Journal and Adveriser* 19 April 1861, 4.
12. *EMJ* 12 (1866-7), 959.
13. *EMJ* 14 (1868-9), pp. 192-3.
14. *Ibid.*
15. Buchan Medical Society minute book, 11 August 1863; 2 August 1864, Aberdeen University Library Manuscripts Collection.
16. Glasgow Southern Medical Society *op.cit.*, minute book, July 4 1850.
17. Glasgow Western Medical Society minute book, 27 February 1908, Library Royal College of Physicians and Surgeons, Glasgow.
18. See for example, Glasgow Southern Medical Society minute book, 20 February 1845, 5 March 1846, Library, Victoria Infirmary, Glasgow.
19. See minute book of the Glasgow Southern Medical Society *op.cit.* 6 March 1851-9 June 1853 *passim.*
20. Aesculapian Club minute book, 17 May 1852, Library Royal College of Physicians, Edinburgh.
21. Aberdeen Medico–Chirurgical Society minute book *op.cit.*, 25 November 1818.
22. *Ibid.*, 5 April 1827.
23. *Ibid.*, 10 October 1848.
24. *Ibid.*, 14 December 1907, 9 January 1908.
25. *Ibid.*, 3 May 1918.
26. *Ibid.*, 3 May 1918.
27. Glasgow Southern Medical Society *op.cit.*, minute book, 16 May 1878.
28. *Ibid.*, 11 October 1888.
29. See for example, minuted meeting of Society held in the Board Room of the Victoria Infirmary, 11 November 1926.
30. Greenock Medico–Chirurgical Association minute book, 10 March 1841, Library Royal College of Physicians and Surgeons, Glasgow.
31. *Ibid.*, 4 May 1841.
32. 'Essays read before the Glasgow Medical Society', Royal College of Physicians and Surgeons of Glasgow Library.
33. See Fife Medico–Chirurgical Society *Circular for the Medical Practitioners of Fife* (Cupar, 1828).
34. 'Essays read before the Glasgow Medical Society' *op.cit.* Vol. 10, Brown 'Remarks on Medical Education', 3 February 1824.
35. *Ibid.*, Vol. 12, Young 'Report of cases admitted at the Eye Infirmary' , 20 December 1825; and Brown 'Observations of some cases in the Medical Wards of the Glasgow Royal Infirmary during the Winter 1824-25', 3 May 1825.
36. *Ibid.*, Robert Perry 'Remarks on Phrenology as connected with the structure of the Brain', 19 April 1825; and Vol. 13 Alexander Hood 'Essay on Phrenology', 7 February 1826.
37. Fife Medico–Chirurgical Society (1828).
38. *Ibid.*
39. *Ibid.*
40. *Ibid.*
41. Cited in MS Presidential Address, 'The Origin of the Garioch and Northern Medical Association' by Dr Peterson for the Society's Jubilee meeting, 1904, among papers of the Society, *op.cit.*
42. Buchan Medical Society minute book *op.cit.*, 11 August 1863.
43. *Ibid.*, 2 August 1864.
44. Garioch and Northern Medical Association, minute book, *op. cit.*, 29 September 1888.
45. The Scottish Midland and Western Medical Association's minute book is held by the present Secretary, Ian Syme, who kindly allowed me access to it in February 1991.

46. SMWMA minute book *op.cit.*, 26 November 1919.
47. *Ibid.*, 29 March 1932.
48. *Ibid.*, 30 July 1873.
49. Clinical Meetings were held at the Royal Infirmary, the Western Infirmary, and the Victoria Infirmary during this year, see Glasgow Southern Medical Society *op. cit.*, minute book 18 February-18 November 1897, *passim*.
50. Glasgow Southern Medical Society *op. cit.*, minute book, 1 April 1926 for note of a visit by the Society to the Cancer Hospital, Hill Street, Glasgow.
51. Handyside 'Address to the Edinburgh Medico-Chirurgical Society' (1874), 783.
52. Dundee Clinical Club *op.cit.*, minute book, 21 July 1894.
53. See Chapter Three, pp. 59–63, for a fuller discussion of the rise of the Edinburgh medical school and the development of the Scottish medical profession.
54. See minutes of the Octogenarian Club, *passim*, Royal College of Physicians of Edinburgh. For more on the Octogenarian Club, see entry 20 in the student and graduate section of Part Two of this book.
55. Granton Club minute book, 2 August 1844, Royal College of Physicians of Edinburgh.
56. See loose MS notes on the history of the Dundee Medical Club, among the Robert Cochrane Buist Papers, Archives Department, University of Dundee.
57. Granton Club minute book *op.cit.* 14 August 1843.
58. The Glasgow Medical Club (1798-1814?) used the system of black-balling candidates from their elite dining club. See Strang (1864), 241-2; 247-51, *passim*.
59. Shepherd (1969), pp. 8-9.
60. *Ibid.*, pp. 56-7.
61. Underhill 'History of the Obstetrical Society of Edinburgh' (1890), 738.
62. Laws of the Edinburgh Obstetrical Society, 18 January 1840, Library of the Royal College of Physicians, Edinburgh.
63. Edinburgh Obstetrical Society *op.cit.* minute book, 13 January 1840.
64. Edinburgh Obstetrical Society *op. cit.*, minute book, 8 December 1840.
65. *Proceedings of the Obstetrical Society of Edinburgh* (Edinburgh, 1847), *passim*.
66. Edinburgh Medico-Chirurgical Society *op.cit.*, minute book, 10 November 1847.
67. Debate on the relative merits of chloroform and ether begun in the middle of the century continued in the Edinburgh Medico-Chirurgical Society in the 1880s. See Report of a meeting of the Society 7 January 1880, *EMJ* 25/2 (1880), 926-34.
68. Report of a meeting of the Edinburgh Medico-Chirurgical Society, 21 November 1849, *Monthly Journal of Medical Science* 10 (1850), 80.
69. Edinburgh Obstetrical Society *op. cit.*, minute book, 25 November 1851, 14 January 1852.
70. Moscucci (1990), 134.
71. *EMJ* 26/2 (Jan-June 1881), 954; see also *EMSJ* 65 (1846), 279 for the original report.
72. See report of 'a case of ovarian disease...' read before the Edinburgh Medico-Chirurgical Society, 3 December 1845 *EMSJ* 65 (1846), 279-308.
73. *Ibid.*, 306.
74. *Ibid.*, 308.
75. Handyside 'Address to the Edinburgh Medico-Chirurgical Society' *EMJ* 19/2 (1874), 1018.
76. *Edinburgh Obstetrical Society Transactions* Vol. 21 (1896), pp. 34-47.
77. *Ibid.*, *passim*.
78. *Ibid.*
79. Park and Daston 'Unnatural Conceptions' (1983), pp. 20-53.
80. *Essays and Observations*, Vol. 2 (1756), v.
81. *Ibid.*, 266.
82. *Ibid.*, pp. 270-2.
83. *Ibid.*, 746.
84. *Ibid.*, 832-3.
85. See Youngson (1979), 155 and *passim*.
86. Underhill 'History of the Obstetrical Society of Edinburgh' (1890), 838.

87. See *Official Year-Book* (1901), 327.
88. *Year-Book, op. cit.*, (1926), 382.
89. *Ibid.*, (1929), 368.
90. *Ibid.*, (1925), 389.
91. *Ibid.*, (1929), 393.
92. Royal Medico-Chirurgical Society of Glasgow printed notice for session 1937-8 pasted into inside cover of minute book, Royal College of Physicians and Surgeons of Glasgow Library.
93. Paper presented at Glasgow Microscopical Society and listed in *Year-Book* (1897), 133.
94. *Ibid.*
95. *Year-Book* (1901), 164.
96. *Ibid.*
97. Figures based on entries for the society listed in the *Year-Book* for these years.
98. Scottish Microscopical Society entry *Year-Book* (1906), 153.
99. Under this heading come papers such as those presented by John Brown Buist, physician and vaccinator at the Western Dispensary, Edinburgh in 1901 on 'The Micro-organisms of Vaccine Materials' and 'On some Recent Advances in our knowledge of Pathogenic Micro-organisms', see *Year-Book* (1901), 162.
100. *Medical Essays* (1733), 297.
101. *Essays and Observations, op. cit., passim.*
102. Edinburgh Obstetrical Society minute book 13 January 1840, Library Royal College of Physicians Edinburgh.
103. *Edinburgh Obstetrical Society Transactions*, Vol. 21 (Edinburgh, 1895), vii.
104. Shepherd *op.cit.*, 42.
105. Simpson (1972), 124.
106. *Ibid.*, 198.
107. *Edinburgh Medico-Chirurgical Society Transactions*, Vol. 3 (1829), *passim.*
108. Edinburgh Medico-Chirurgical Society *op.cit.*, Council minute book, 27 January 1903.
109. For more on the Scottish branches of the Medical Women's Federation see Chapter Five, pp. 96–7.
110. Medical Women's Federation Archives, Mabel Rew 'Notes on the Medical Women's Federation' Jubilee Meeting, 1967, Wellcome Institute for the History of Medicine, London Contemporary Archives Centre.
111. Medical Women's Federation Archives *op.cit.*, Annie Gillie, MS notes of the history of the Medical Women's Federation, 12 November 1954.

CHAPTER THREE

The Formation of the Professional Elite and Scottish Medical Societies

The first two chapters of this work have described the basic nature, distribution, activities, and concerns, of Scottish medical societies in the period 1731-1939. This chapter and the following two aim to provide a more interpretative framework with which to assess the role of the societies in the development of the medical profession in Scotland. This chapter, in particular, is concerned with the intellectual and organisational background to professional development and society formation in the eighteenth century, when clubs and societies consisted chiefly of the Edinburgh-based elite of the profession, who were members of the colleges of physicians and surgeons. Later societies were more broadly based. The formation of medical societies in Scotland in the eighteenth century is an integral part of the development of the medical profession in this period of the Scottish Enlightenment, most often measured by the establishment of the medical faculty of the University of Edinburgh and the setting-up of student teaching facilities in the recently-opened Royal Infirmary in the city. A mutual intellectual endeavour lay behind the formation of the early medical societies and the provision of medical education in Edinburgh, indeed, it is often possible to identify common personnel in these activities. The focus on Edinburgh for most of the discussion of eighteenth-century Scottish medicine is due to the unique set of circumstances which allowed the city to lead the way in medical education and medical science.

EARLY HISTORY OF THE MEDICAL PROFESSION IN SCOTLAND COMPARED WITH ENGLAND

It is a commonly accepted view[1] that the practice of medicine in pre-industrial British society was divided into three orders, each with its own standing in the wider community. This stratification of medical practice into physician, surgeon, and apothecary, was compounded by the existence of six medical corporations, three in England and three in Scotland. In England these were the Royal College of Physicians (1518); the Company of Surgeons (which until 1745 was associated with the barbers from its foundation in 1540, and became the Royal College of Surgeons of London in 1800); and the Worshipful Society of Apothecaries (1617). In Scotland there were the Incorporation of Surgeons and Barbers of Edinburgh (1505), which became the College of Surgeons in 1726; the Faculty of Physicians and Surgeons in Glasgow (1599); and the College of Physicians of Edinburgh (1681). Thus, Scotland did not mirror the tripartite division in England and a more cohesive medical profession emerged earlier in Scotland. Physicians and surgeons belonged to the same medical faculty in Glasgow from the late sixteenth century, while in Edinburgh the fusion of apothecaries' and surgeons' duties was completed by 1656.[2]

The Glasgow Faculty of Physicians and Surgeons provided diplomas for graduate physicians, and instruction and examination in anatomy, surgery, botany and pharmacy for its surgeon members. A similar pattern of licensed recognition of physicians' university qualifications (graduates who did not possess a degree from a Scottish University were required to pass an examination to test their knowledge) and examinations of surgeons' competency was repeated in the Edinburgh colleges of physicians and surgeons respectively. In both Edinburgh and Glasgow attendance at University medical classes was used to foreshorten the period of apprenticeship in surgery, which was usually of five years' duration. As well as granting licences and diplomas to duly qualified practitioners, the Colleges aimed to exclude 'irregular' practitioners from the areas within their jurisdiction. For much of the eighteenth and nineteenth centuries, the monthly meetings of the Glasgow Faculty included hearings of 'irregulars' summoned to appear before the Faculty for unlicensed practice, some of whom admitted their offence and signed undertakings not to practise or risk incurring a fine;[3] others on examination were admitted to the Faculty,[4] while the majority probably refused to attend the Faculty hearings or went completely undetected.

The three Scottish medical corporations were not concerned simply with the regulation of medical practice in their areas. All three became involved in the provision of free vaccination services for the local poor. Inoculation against smallpox was promoted jointly by the Edinburgh Colleges in 1791, although it was the surgeons who undertook the actual vaccination.[5] In Glasgow, the Faculty ran a 'vaccination station' for the poor in the city throughout the nineteenth century,[6] and frequently provided free attendance for the 'deserving poor' recommended by local churches and public authorities.[7]

Despite the wide base for medical training available in Scotland in the medical corporations, their role in professional development is not clear-cut. In fact, all three groups, the two Edinburgh Colleges and the Glasgow Faculty, on occasion came into conflict with each other, and, in the case of the Glasgow Faculty in the years 1826–40, with the city's University, over issues of professional jurisdiction and education.

> There was opposition to the development of university medical teaching by the Faculty of Physicians and Surgeons who felt that they alone should supervise the training of surgeons and the licensing of physicians in Glasgow.[8]

Much earlier, at the end of the seventeenth century, the Edinburgh Incorporation of Surgeons tried desperately to prevent the formation of a college of physicians, as a threat to their own position.

On hearing of the intention of the physicians to seek incorporation, the surgeons nominated a committee of sixteen members to oppose it with all their might, being afraid that if the Charter were granted 'it might mightily encroach upon their privileges....'[9]

There were occasions when the two Edinburgh Colleges and the Glasgow Faculty combined, but these were generally provoked by external threats to Scottish practitioners and the integrity of the Colleges themselves, and it was not until the end of the nineteenth century that the long-standing animosity between the two Edinburgh Colleges was finally removed, with the setting up of a School of Medicine of the Royal Colleges of Edinburgh in 1895, a consequence of the changes in the structure of medical education wrought by the passage of the 1886 Medical Act Amendment Act. The school lasted until the National Health Service reforms of 1948.[10]

Although the emphasis so far in this chapter has been on the regulation of 'qualified' practitioners, 'non-qualified' or 'irregular' practitioners and druggists provided the main source of medical relief for the vast majority of British society until well into the nineteenth century. Indeed, one inquiry in 1805 revealed that unqualified practitioners outnumbered their qualified counterparts in the order of 9 to 1.[11] This group ought not to be regarded simply as being made up of 'quacks' preying on an innocent population with their outrageous claims for the cure-all propensities of patent remedies: among this section of the medical population were included bone-setters, folk healers, homoeopaths, and most significantly, midwives, all of whom had contributions to make towards the provision of medical care. The frequent outbursts of the regular medical practitioners against 'quackery' were not due only to the numbers of those involved in 'irregular' practice, but also owed much to the intense competition for patients within the expanding ranks of 'regular' medicine.

The Scottish medical corporations were in a sense, the earliest forms of professional association. Yet, in the course of the eighteenth century, their hierarchical, elitist structure increasingly presented a challenge to the developing profession, as represented by the newly formed medical clubs and societies. 'The exclusiveness, selfishness, and slothfulness of their fossilized corporations were the target of reformers for more than half a century after the new wave of association had set in.'[12] Although first expressed in clubs and societies formed by the elite of the profession, these newly-formed groups were established on cross-corporate lines, and tended towards cohesion rather than at maintaining status-based division in the profession. The tendency to equality within the profession may be first seen in the contributors to the *Medical Essays and Observations* of the Edinburgh Medical Society. Two of the five volumes contained the same number of attributable papers by physicians and surgeons, and on the occasions when there was an imbalance in the number of essays included by physicians and surgeons, as in the final volume where there were thirteen papers contributed by physicians and 26 by surgeons, this was caused by the large number of contributions from Alexander Monro *primus*, who had ten essays in the final volume of the *Medical Essays*.[13] Of course, status-based division was not removed between physicians and surgeons overnight. Reference to the membership list of the Edinburgh Philosophical Society for 1739 shows eight physicians to four surgeons in the ranks of this elite society.[14] The best example of the attempt to overcome the divisions between physicians and surgeons in the city can be found in the formation of the Aesculapian Club set up in 1773 by Andrew Duncan.[15]

> The main object of the Club... was, to cement the friendship between the two Royal Colleges, of Physicians and Surgeons. Accordingly, the first regulation reads: 'The Club shall consist of twenty-two members, chosen from among the Fellows of the Colleges of Physicians and Surgeons'. Although the number from each College has never been fixed by any rule, it has remained equal or nearly equal for almost two centuries.[16]

Despite such attempts to overcome professional divisions, the medical community in Edinburgh was still dominated by an elite: the Aesculapian Club was strictly limited in the size of its membership, potential new members were balloted for and one black ball was sufficient for rejection.[17] The medical corporations also maintained their elite nature. An increasingly common area of complaint in the course of the eighteenth and nineteenth centuries was the exorbitant level of fees charged by the Scottish corporations for membership. This was due to the compulsory obligation of members of each medical corporation to join the widows' fund; a necessary, but expensive form of mutual insurance given the relatively high mortality rates for practitioners, particularly during times of epidemic fever. By the middle of the nineteenth century the cost of joining the Royal College of Surgeons of Edinburgh was £250, half of which went straight into the widows' fund,[18] while in Glasgow the cost of Faculty membership was £150, two-thirds of which subsidised the widows' fund.[19] The detrimental effect of such high fees was felt in the declining number of practitioners enrolling in the Scottish corporations. This trend continued despite the institution of lesser licentiate memberships. Licentiateships were introduced to avoid the high cost of joining the widows' funds but excluded the new category of members from all voting rights and participation in corporate activities. This lesser category of corporate membership was devised to boost the enrolment figures of the Scottish corporations after a century of spiralling fees, and within the space of a year (1850–1), both the RCSE and the FPSG resorted to Act of Parliament to amend their charters and remove the compulsory widows' fund contribution from the cost of membership.[20]

The reduction in the numbers enrolling in the Scottish corporations due to the high cost of membership aptly illustrates the limits of their jurisdiction. Until the passage of the 1858 Medical Act, there was no legal requirement for medical practitioners in Scotland to register their qualifications (let alone a legal restriction on unqualified medical practice), nor indeed, was any medical qualification required in areas outside the jurisdiction of the corporations, which for the College of Surgeons was the city of Edinburgh, the Lothians, Fife and parts of the Borders.[21] The Glasgow Faculty's jurisdiction covered the city, Lanark, Renfrew, Ayrshire and Dumbarton.[22] The most restricted jurisdiction was that of the Edinburgh College of Physicians, which was limited to Edinburgh and its suburbs.[23]

The divisions, costs and restricted jurisdiction of the Scottish medical corporations meant that although they were based on a broader system of medical instruction and examination than was the case in England, the traditional position of the Scottish corporations, enjoyed since the sixteenth century, was gradually undermined. The challenge arose from an increasingly university-based system of medical education, and the emergence of a more cohesive, although admittedly still somewhat elite, group of medical practitioners who increasingly in the eighteenth century formed their own professional societies and clubs outside the rigid, divisive confines of the medical corporations.

MEDICAL ETHICS

The formation of medical societies was the method of professional self-regulation increasingly adopted by medical practitioners in the course of the late eighteenth and early nineteenth centuries, as in the setting up of the Aesculapian Club and Harveian Society in Edinburgh. One of the chief concerns of the new organisations was to regulate intra-professional relationships, in order to create unity and cooperation within the group. The way to achieve this ideal was through the formation of ethical codes.

The starting point for any analysis of medical ethics in this period must be Thomas Percival's seminal work *Medical Ethics*, published in Manchester in 1803. This book had a profound effect, both on contemporary and later medical practitioners, and has had an integral part to play in the works of countless medical historians addressing the issue of the development of the medical profession in Britain. Percival's work was prompted by an intra-professional dispute between staff at Manchester's Royal Infirmary in the early 1790s, which Percival (as physician extraordinary) was asked to resolve by drawing up a code of conduct for the staff. This work was published privately in 1794, nine years before its general release. Percival's work, although deriving from a specific situation, had a widespread application. In it, he sought to maintain the tripartite division of the medical profession. The fact that in this Percival was fighting a losing battle does not lessen the value of his work, particularly bearing in mind that it was written in the early 1790s, suggesting that the old divisions of medicine were increasingly being undermined by this time.

Percival's work was important for the general professionalisation of medicine. He advances the cause of friendly and professional intercourse, to promote understanding and knowledge within the profession; likewise, he suggested that common fees should be established on a local basis,[24] and he warned against the dangers of criticising or belittling the common body of medical men:

A physician ... should cautiously guard against whatever may injure the

Figure 3.1: Front page of a report on medical ethics by the North of Scotland Medical Association, 1872.

REPORT

OF THE

COMMITTEE ON "MEDICAL ETHICS"

APPOINTED BY

The North of Scotland Medical Association,

JULY, 1871.

AT INVERURIE, 8*th June,* 1872.

YOUR Committee had under consideration the remit made to them at last Annual Meeting, and Resolution by the Garioch and Northern Medical Association, recommending 'the Compilation of a Code of Ethics to their careful diligence,' also copies of the Rules of the Manchester and of the York Medico-Ethical Association; and having carefully considered these and the whole question, recommend the following as the basis of such a Code.

GEORGE MACKIE, *Convener.*

1.—A Gentleman commencing the practice of his profession will be expected to introduce himself by calling on those medical men who may be in the district or neighbourhood. And it will be their duty to return his visit by extending to him the ordinary courtesies of society.

2.—Unless introduced to the practice of another, or where there is no other practitioner in the district, the person commencing practice will be expected to *wait* for those who may wish to consult him. And on no account will it be considered gentlemanly conduct to seek, by personal visiting or otherwise, interest and employment in the district.

3.—When during sickness, affliction, or absence from home, a practitioner has entrusted the care of his patients (or practice) to a professional friend, the person so entrusted shall not make any charge on the patients for his services, but shall simply be the *Locum Teneus* of the absentee.

4.—When a Practitioner is called in a case of emergency, to a family usually attended by another, so soon as the emergency is provided for, he shall, unless *specially* requested to continue attendance, resign the case into the hands of the ordinary attendant of the family, but shall be entitled to his fee.

5.—When a Practitioner is waited on for consultation, or requested to visit a patient whom he has previously attended as the *Locum Teneus* of a friend during his sickness or absence from home, it will be the duty of that Practitioner *to decline*.

Reproduced by kind permission of the Archivist, Aberdeen University Manuscripts Collection.

general respectability of his profession; and should avoid all... jocularity or scepticism, concerning the efficacy and utility of the healing art.[25]

Percival's *Medical Ethics* exercised great influence on the ethical input into the growing number of local medical societies,[26] which groups were to become such a feature of medical development in the eighteenth and nineteenth centuries. The question which has occupied some medical historians, of whether Percival's work dealt with medical 'ethics' or simply professional medical 'etiquette', is largely a question of semantics. Both terms in their dictionary sense can be proffered as descriptions of Percival's code, and the assumption that only 'doctor–patient' relationships are the true ground for the exercise of 'medical ethics', appears to be too narrow a definition.[27]

The cause of intra-professional conflict, initially played out in the ranks of the medical corporations, and later in the challenge of university medical faculties and local societies to the corporations, was not simply the erosion of the old divisions in medical practice which left medical practitioners unsure of their respective positions and status in society: it was also due to the increased competition between medical men as the profession expanded. From these feelings of insecurity and fierce competition grew the local medical societies, and later national societies.[28] Hand in hand with the rise in medical organisation went the campaign for the reform of medical education and the regularisation of medical practice: the professional and medico-political issues which played an increasingly important role in medical societies.

EDINBURGH MEDICINE AND EIGHTEENTH–CENTURY MEDICAL SOCIETIES

Although some reference was made to early Scottish medical societies in the opening two chapters, these first examples of professional association are deserving of closer attention for their close links with the rise of Edinburgh medical science and education in the course of the eighteenth century. The history of clubs and societies in eighteenth century Edinburgh is a well-worn path,[29] particularly for historians of science.[30] However, the specifically medical societies have never been examined as constituting a separate entity. This is understandable, since although these unions of individual medical practitioners suggest the early advance of the professionalisation process among Scottish medical elites, medical society formation cannot be considered in isolation. The individuals most involved in this new form of medical cooperation and education can also be identified with the emerging ruling order in Edinburgh 'polite' society from the 1720s onwards, and more generally, with the emergence of Edinburgh medicine as a key intellectual element in the Scottish Enlightenment.

While not wishing to identify the development of Edinburgh medicine too closely with one individual, it is clear that Alexander Monro *primus*,[31] (first Professor of Anatomy at Edinburgh University) as well as playing an integral part in the formation of the University's Medical Faculty, was also instrumental in establishing the earliest medical society for which documentation exists in Scotland: the Edinburgh Medical Society, formed in 1731. The Society was not created in a vacuum, however, since medical and other, broader-based scientific clubs had existed in Edinburgh in the late seventeenth and early eighteenth centuries in a more limited form, and at least five were set up in the twenty years after 1684.[32] The vital difference between these earlier medical and/or scientific clubs and the Edinburgh Medical Society (itself formed shortly after the creation of the Medical Faculty and the opening of the Royal Infirmary in the city) lies in the fact that the EMS was formed expressly for the purpose of producing a publication devoted to the furtherance of medical knowledge.

Monro *primus* was the dominating force behind the Society, both in terms of his extensive contributions, and editorial control. A contemporary manuscript, most likely by Monro himself, gives the impression that the society very quickly became a one-man production.

> During the first year the members attended the monthly meetings of the society, and made remarks on the papers read to them. But after the publication of their first volume in 1732 [sic], they neglected attendance, and the whole care of the collection was taken by the Secretary [Monro] without any other member seeing any of the papers except what some of them were authors of till after they were printed.[33]

Largely following this information, Emerson, in the first of his series of articles on the Philosophical Society, sees Monro *primus* as the personification of the Medical Society.

> From 1732 to 1737 Monro embodied the Society, collecting its papers, editing them, and seeing through the press volumes in 1733, 1734, 1735 and 1737. If the Society did not thrive, it certainly appeared healthy and flourishing to an increasing number of British and European medical men who read its works, not only in English, but also in the French translations which began to appear in 1733. Its health however, was contingent upon Monro's, and this failed in about 1736.[34]

It is clear that the influence and importance of the Edinburgh Medical Society of 1731 to 1737 stretched beyond its relatively short life span, and its apparent dominance by one individual. Its existence serves to highlight the close connection between the rise of the Edinburgh Medical Faculty, the Royal Infirmary, and the organised profession. Even although it had ceased to be, in any practical sense, a 'society', within a year, it did mark the beginning of a trend in medical cooperation in which the correspondent of a medical society/journal was provided with both a forum and a focus for medical debate and education, a fact which remains vital in the continued existence of periodical publications up to the present time. Indeed, the more general role of the written communication to a society is something which is important, providing as it does, a network of contact far exceeding the geographical limits of a society's regular attendance, at a time when organized transport between cities was both irregular and hazardous.

The Edinburgh Medical Society's network of correspondents stretched across Scotland and to parts of England and Ireland, but its influence can be measured in terms of the whole continent of Europe, particularly at a time when access to books on medical topics was by no means widespread. In this way the section in each of the five volumes, (part 2 in volume 5), containing the list of books published on medical matters was an integral part of the improvement of medical knowledge, which was the avowed purpose of the *Medical Essays*, and the society which spawned them.

The work of the Edinburgh Medical Society was continued in the printed proceedings of the Edinburgh Philosophical Society, 1737–83, which despite its name and avowed intentions to improve the level of knowledge in both arts and science, remained largely a medical society, with the majority of its printed transactions, and at its close, the majority of its members, medical in character. The main difference between the two societies was the presence in the ranks of the Philosophical Society of the non-medical elite, patrons of the arts and sciences, who added prestige to the society. Somewhat ironically, the decline of the Philosophical Society was linked to the success of another periodical publication, Andrew Duncan senior's *Medical Commentaries* first published in 1773.[35] The regular volumes of *Commentaries* provided a more successful alternative to the infrequently published transactions, and a decade later the Philosophical Society was replaced by the broader-based Royal Society of Edinburgh.

The emergence of the Edinburgh Medical Society in the 1730s was due in part to the unique educational and economic circumstances then prevailing in Edinburgh. Historians have identified the crucial role of the Town Council in the creation and expansion of the Medical Faculty at Edinburgh.[36] Edinburgh Town Council was unique in Scotland in its control over the local University, and its dominance by merchant and trading guilds saw the provision of medical education in a similar vein. Based on local economic considerations the Town Council's support for the expansion of the University's Medical Faculty ensured enthusiastic local Scottish attendance and attracted other British and overseas students to the city.[37]

Local factors stressed by Shapin in the development of University medical education also help to explain why it was Edinburgh and not Glasgow or Aberdeen, which witnessed the origin, and later, proliferation, of medical societies in the eighteenth century. This is not to suggest however, that these cities had no influence on the development of medical thought and education during the century. There were papers from two Glasgow surgeons in the first volume of the *Medical Essays*, while John Paisley, another Glasgow surgeon, had papers in all the subsequent volumes, and was to be an original member of the Philosophical Society of Edinburgh in 1737, alongside John Johnston, the titular Professor of Medicine at Glasgow University.[38] But, while John Paisley lectured extra-murally in Glasgow on Anatomy, Johnston is unlikely to have delivered a course of lectures during his tenure of office as Professor of Medicine, indicating the somnolent state of University medical teaching in Glasgow at this time.[39] The slow progress in the development of University-based medical education in Glasgow, independent of external motivating agencies such as the Town Council and without an infirmary for student instruction until 1794, also helps to explain why it lagged behind Edinburgh in the development of medical and other scientific societies.

It has been argued that the difference between Glasgow and Edinburgh in the fifty years between 1780 and 1830 in the history of science was due to the fact that, in Glasgow, businessmen (merchants and manufacturers), were more prominent than professionals, while the position was reversed in Edinburgh. The difference is reflected in the contrast between the membership of the Glasgow Philosophical Society (established in 1802), with that of the Edinburgh Royal Society (established in 1783). Manufacturers, artisans and merchants made up the majority of the former, while the latter contained a cross-section of the Edinburgh elite; mainly professors, medical men, lawyers and gentry.[40] It is probable that this lack of prominence among the professions in Glasgow dates back earlier in the eighteenth century, and is in sharp contrast to the developments in Edinburgh. There was, however, a forum for wide-ranging intellectual debate in existence in Glasgow in the mid-eighteenth century in the shape of the Literary Society, formed in 1755, which discussed scientific topics, including medical subjects.[41]

In Aberdeen, two of the six founding members of the city's Philosophical Society established in 1754, were medical men, and there were a number of medical contributions to the society's proceedings. But this society remained a small group, and as with its Glasgow counter-part lacked the sustained impetus towards educational enterprise and professional cooperation provided by the Faculty of Medicine at Edinburgh.[42]

The influence of the local economic and educational factors existing in Edinburgh from the 1720s cannot be over-stressed when analysing the rise of the medical profession in the city, including the emergence of medical societies and clubs. From the beginning made by the Edinburgh Medical Society in 1731, later-eighteenth century associations of the medical elite were formed in the city.[43] These groups were more limited, and of a chiefly convivial nature: the most prominent were the Aesculapian Club (1773), the Harveian Society (1782), and the Gymnastic Society (1786). These clubs formed by Andrew Duncan Senior were intended to bring physicians and surgeons together in an atmosphere of fraternity, and to help overcome self-interested professional division. The Aesculapian Club has already been mentioned, while the Gymnastic Society was its sporting off-shoot. The Harveian Society was first mooted as a larger version of the Aesculapian, formed to take over the burden of running the Aesculapian's prize medical essay competition, which with its five guinea award was proving too expensive for the limited membership of the older Club to maintain.[44]

The creation of convivial societies for Edinburgh physicians and surgeons in the late eighteenth century counter-balanced the continuing struggle between the two rival corporations in the city. Until the beginning of the nineteenth century, the physicians successfully opposed the institution of a chair in Surgery at the University, and the surgeons were further alienated after 1785 by their exclusion from the nominations for honorary appointments in the Royal Infirmary. Indeed, during the late 1780s many prominent surgeons in the city resigned from their Infirmary duties, and by the turn of the century only four of the twenty three senior surgeons on the roll of the Royal College of Surgeons remained attached to the Infirmary.[45] Such evidence would seem to suggest that the elite of the Scottish medical profession, far from being cohesive, was in reality bitterly divided between physicians and surgeons. However, at the same time as corporate division in Edinburgh was so forcefully demonstrated, medical clubs and societies attempted to overcome such tension and allow physicians and surgeons to meet together in a fraternal atmosphere.

The intellectual advance of Edinburgh medicine in many related spheres in the course of the eighteenth century was the leading factor in the process of professionalisation in the practice of medicine across Scotland in this period. Although these activities may have been at first chiefly confined to the elite of the profession, it was not necessarily bound to the geographical limits of Edinburgh due to the influence of, and contributions to, the variety of printed transactions discussed earlier. Intellectual endeavour in the University Medical Faculty, in the Royal Infirmary, in medical clubs and societies, and in published transactions, did not simply speed the professionalisation of Scottish medicine, but also, to a great extent, shaped the scientific input of the Scottish Enlightenment. The Royal Medical Society of Edinburgh provides an example.

THE ROYAL MEDICAL SOCIETY OF EDINBURGH

The history of the 'student' Royal Medical Society cannot be divorced from a discussion of eighteenth century medical societies, although students were not a recognised part of the elite of the profession. However, the student body was a powerful independent institution due to the peculiar structure of the Edinburgh Medical School, which gave students great freedom of choice in class selection. It was from student fees that the professoriate and extra-mural lecturers derived a substantial amount of their income, and they therefore were of necessity forced to pay heed to the students' opinions.[46] In addition, eighteenth-century Edinburgh student medical societies were characterised by their 'freedom of spirit':

> The medical societies of students, which have been conducted with decency and regularity, have in this, as well as in other respects, produced the best effects. In these, they have been taught to feel and exercise their own powers, to arrange their ideas, and to express them with facility...[47]

For much of the eighteenth century at least, those 'students' who made up the majority of the membership of the RMS were often already graduates in other subjects. Some had also already engaged in medical practice, and came to study medicine in Edinburgh to further their education. As the reputation of the Medical Faculty rose it drew to it those who wished to augment their medical knowledge and increase their prestige, not necessarily immediately sitting for their MD in doing so. The example of the early career of William Cullen is a case in point. After serving a two-year apprenticeship to a Glasgow surgeon, Cullen acted as a ship's surgeon on a two year voyage to the West Indies. Only after a further year in practice did he, in 1734, proceed to Edinburgh University to study medicine. In 1735, he joined the medical society which was to become the Royal Medical Society two years later. In 1736, he left to set up a new practice in Hamilton, and eventually took his MD at Glasgow University in 1740.[48]

The pattern of Cullen's early career suggests that it would be inaccurate to categorise the Royal Medical Society as a 'student society' at a time when the achievement of an MD was not the first priority of a medical practitioner. This is further highlighted in the case of Alexander Monro *secundus*, who became conjoint Professor of Anatomy and Surgery with his father in 1754, when he had no formal medical qualifications (although he had previously studied mathematics and philosophy at the University), and was aged only 21.[49] There were also a number of practitioners who remained active in the society after qualification; four, including Andrew Duncan senior, are referred to in the Society's minute book for 1780,[50] while in a unique bound volume of papers read to the society in 1779-80, five of the twelve contributors had already qualified.[51]

Under the direct influence of former student members, including Cullen and Duncan senior, who became lecturers in Edinburgh, the Society came to challenge prevailing medical orthodoxy.[52] In fact, the Royal Medical Society in the late eighteenth century became the focus of intellectual discussion and debate outside the fixed structures of the profession. The best example of the critical function of members of the RMS on medical orthodoxy is to be found in the heated debates within the Society over the merits of the Brunonian system during the 1770s and 1780s. John Brown, an extra-mural lecturer in Edinburgh, put forward a theory that good health was maintained by a series of stimuli, including alcohol and opium, which were to be liberally administered to engender the correct degree of excitability.[53]

The close connection between the activities of the RMS and contemporary medical thought in the University and extra-mural schools is apparent when it is noted that it was in the discussions of the Society that the Brunonian system fought for credibility.

> When his [Brown's] application for the Chair of the Institutes of Medicine proved unsuccessful, he began, in 1778, to deliver lectures on his new system, using the manuscript of his *Elementa Medicinae* as his text-book. The students formed two parties, the Cullenians and the Brunonians, and debated the points at issue with partisan heat; the latter, as rebels against authority, showed the greater vehemence in the very lively debates at the meetings of the Royal Medical Society.[54]

The friction caused by the partisan debate ultimately led to the resignation of one of Brown's supporters, John Richard Martyn from the Society; tendered rather than face expulsion for, among other things, 'attempt[ing]... to introduce new modes of settling differences in debate by appeals to the sword...'.[55] It was also apparently he who leaked biased reports of the Society's meetings to the *Edinburgh Evening Post* which led to a court action by the RMS.[56] His letter of resignation makes clear the bitter intellectual divisions between the supporters of Cullen and those of Brown, as he refers to:

> some Despotic Teachers whose prejudice and self interest are a sufficient reason for them to do everything in their favour for their own ends to keep students in the Dark that the fallacy of their own Doctrine may not appear, from the evident superiority of a Doctrine [Brunonianism] founded on the simple laws of animal oeconomy and the Dictates of common sense...[57]

The Royal Medical Society in the course of the eighteenth century provided an extended platform for medical discussion in Edinburgh, outside the elitist confines of the University Medical Faculty and the medical corporations. It has been suggested that support for Brunonianism also, '... indicated there was room in the Edinburgh educational market-place for competition from new ideas and approaches different to those associated with the Edinburgh professoriate'.[58] The heated debate played out in the ranks of the 'student' body, albeit under the influence of their instructors, provides evidence of the inter-dependence of the intellectual medical community in the city during the eighteenth century. It also provides evidence to suggest that medical clubs and societies in the eighteenth century were not simply smooth-running social organisations, scientific and professional disputes surfaced in these groups as in other fields of medical contact.

For most of the eighteenth century Scottish intellectual medical activity was focused on the profession in Edinburgh due to a unique combination of circumstances, including the interventionist support of the Town Council, and the emergence of figures such as Monro *primus* and Duncan senior. Their influence was felt across the whole spectrum of medical intellectual activity: from the creation of the Medical Faculty of Edinburgh University, to the opening of the Royal Infirmary; from the setting up of medical periodicals, to the formation of clubs and societies. However, the institutional basis for such activity ensured that professional development tended to remain in the hands of the Edinburgh medical elite for much of the century.

It is clear that medical societies form an integral part of the intellectual make-up of Scottish medicine. They were also to the fore in much medico-political and professional debate. In spanning these areas medical societies provide a unique link between the concerns of the eighteenth century elite of the profession and those of more interest to the rank and file of the profession which form the mainstay of the next two chapters.

NOTES

1. See for example Parry (1976); Peterson (1978); Waddington (1984), *passim.*
2. Comrie (1927), 183.
3. Duncan (1896), 94.
4. *Ibid.*, 160.
5. Craig (1976), pp. 181–2.
6. Duncan (1896), pp. 153–5.
7. *Ibid.*, 94.
8. Hamilton (1981), 125.
9. Creswell (1926), 119.
10. *Ibid.*, 344.
11. Newman (1957), 59.
12. Carr-Saunders and Wilson (1930), 300.
13. See *Medical Essays* Vol. 5 (1737), *passim.*
14. Edinburgh Philosophical Society (1737), pp. 13–14.
15. For biographical details of Andrew Duncan senior see Chapter One, pp. 12–13.
16. Guthrie, 'Aesculapian Club' (1967), 245.
17. *Ibid.*, 246.
18. Creswell (1926), 276.
19. Duncan (1896), 159.
20. See Creswell (1926), 277, and Duncan (1896), 159.
21. Creswell *op.cit.*, pp. 121–2.
22. Craig (1976), 144.
23. *Ibid.*
24. Percival (1827), 326.
25. *Ibid.*, pp. 226–7.
26. See Chapter Two, pp. 33–4, for further reference to the ethical discussions of some of the Scottish societies.
27. Waddington 'Development of Medical Ethics' (1975), 40, has argued that most ethical debates of the period revolved along professional competitive lines, rather than doctor–patient relationships, 'Virtually all of the literature from this period supports the idea that relationships between practitioners were much more in need of regulation, than were relationships between practitioners and their patients'.
28. The Provincial Medical and Surgical Association was set up in 1832 and in 1855 became the British Medical Association. For more on the BMA see Chapter Five, pp. 79–82, 97–103.
29. The trend began with McElroy's 'Literary Clubs and Societies of 18th Century Scotland' (1952). See also McElroy (1969) *passim.*
30. See in particular, Emerson's series of four articles on 'The Philosophical Society of Edinburgh', (1979), 154–91; (1981), 133–76; (1985), 255–303; (1988), 33–66, and Morrell 'University of Edinburgh in the late eighteenth century' (1971), 158–71; and 'Reflections on the history of Scottish science' (1974), 95–121.
31. For more on the life of Alexander Monro *primus*, see Wright-St.Clair (1964), *passim.*
32. Emerson, 'Science and the Origins and Concerns of the Scottish Enlightenment' (1988), 353.
33. *Ibid.*
34. Emerson, 'Philosophical Society of Edinburgh 1737–1747' (1979), 158.
35. Emerson, 'Philosophical Society of Edinburgh 1768–1783' (1985), pp. 266–7.
36. Chitnis, 'Provost Drummond and the Origins of Edinburgh Medicine', ch. in Campbell and Skinner (1982), 91.
37. Shapin, 'Audience for Science in 18th Century Edinburgh' (1974), 97.
38. *Regulations of the Edinburgh Philosophical Society of Edinburgh op.cit.*, 14.
39. Comrie (1927), pp. 357–9 *passim.*
40. Morrell, 'Reflections on the History of Scottish Science' (1974), 80.
41. Emerson, 'Science and the Origins and Concerns of the Scottish Enlightenment' (1985), 365, n. 106.

42. Ulman (1990), 21.
43. See Appendix 2 for a chronological list of student clubs and societies set up in Scotland.
44. Innes, 'Harveians of Edinburgh' (1983), 285.
45. Risse (1986), 65.
46. Lawrence, 'Medicine as Culture' (1984), 196.
47. Gregory (1772), 7.
48. Comrie (1927), 311.
49. Wright-St. Clair (1964), 70.
50. Royal Medical Society minute book, 1780, *passim*, RMS library, 22 Bristo Square, Edinburgh University.
51. See Edinburgh [Royal] Medical Society, Papers read to the Society, 1779–80, library, Royal College of Physicians of Edinburgh.
52. Lawrence (1984), 205.
53. Gray (1952), 51. For recent discussions on the influence of Brown's thinking, see Bynum and Porter (1988), *passim*.
54. Gray (1952), 52.
55. Royal Medical Society minute book *op.cit.*, 10 February. 1781.
56. *Ibid.*, pp. 57–8.
57. *Ibid.*, 12 February 1781.
58. Barfoot, 'Brunonianism under the bed' ch. in Bynum and Porter (1988), 44.

CHAPTER FOUR

The Disreputable and the Contentious: 'Resurrectionism' and Phrenology in Medical Society Debate

The origins and activities of the first Scottish medical societies and clubs reflected the development of the Scottish medical profession in the eighteenth century. Yet not all Scottish medical intellectual involvement fits into the traditional picture of 'progressive' scientific and educational endeavour dominated by the professional elite. By way of contrast to the previous one, this chapter highlights two areas where various elements of the Scottish medical profession were active in matters of problematic medical concern in the course of the first half of the nineteenth century: 'resurrectionism' and phrenology. The Royal Medical Society's debates on ambiguous medical thought in the shape of Brunonianism just mentioned moves the discussion away from a consideration of elite medical intellectual activity centred on Edinburgh. Brown's theory of stimulation illuminate the contentious aspects of medical intellectual involvement and the problematic nature of 'orthodox' medical knowledge. In the case of 'resurrectionism', or body-snatching, disreputable practice was used to pursue a proper medico-scientific goal - anatomical investigation. Also in the first half of the nineteenth century, elements of the medical profession in Scotland pursued the science of phrenology, and the medical societies reflected this trend.

RESURRECTIONISM

The protracted dispute over resurrectionism is an area which helps bring into focus the problems facing the profession across Scotland for much of the early part of the nineteenth century, as it sought to achieve a recognised status among the wider community. Both the Royal Medical Society and the Aberdeen Medical Society (later reconstituted as the Aberdeen Medico-Chirurgical Society), discussed the contentious subject of resurrectionism and its repercussions for the medical profession.

Resurrectionism was an issue which came to provoke much professional discussion and public outcry in the first three decades of the nineteenth century. Within the profession, debate on this problematic subject was conducted in the ranks of medical societies. Controversy over anatomical supplies had been an issue for much of the eighteenth century too; in 1725, there was an attack on Monro *primus*' anatomy theatre (he was city Professor of Anatomy after 1722) by a crowd angry at alleged body-snatching for use in his classes.[1] In 1749, most of the windows of the Faculty of Physicians and Surgeons in Glasgow were smashed by a crowd after a rumour spread that one of the city's graveyards had been violated by body-snatchers.[2]

The two Scottish societies most closely involved with the issue of anatomical reform and the difficulty of ensuring a regular supply of subjects were the Royal Medical Society, and the Aberdeen Medical (later Medico-Chirurgical) Society, both of which had a strong 'student' representation. In 1828, the Royal Medical Society petitioned parliament on the subject of anatomy reform, in terms which virtually admitted their complicity in the activities of resurrectionists:

> ... your petitioners respectfully approach your honourable House to lay before your Lordships a statement of the difficulties under which they as members of the medical profession[3] labour in the acquisition of a most important branch of their professional knowledge... in their endeavours to attain the requisite information, they are visited with prosecution and actually subjected to fines and imprisonment.[4]

Two years later, and after the great controversy caused in the city by the body-procuring activities of Burke and Hare, the Society again petitioned parliament, although this time the tone of their petition was much less complacent:

> The members of the Medical Profession are entirely dependent for the means of anatomical knowledge on the exertions of certain individuals, who, from the exposure of the horrible atrocities disclosed on the trial of William Burke have proved themselves capable of committing the most revolting crimes to obtain the supply of subjects required by the schools of anatomy.
>
> That deeply impressed with a sense of the evils arising out of this state of things... your petitioners would, with much anxiety... press upon the attention of your honourable House the necessity that exists for the introduction of some measure by which the attainment of subjects for dissection may be legalised, and thus at once the violation of the sepulchre be prevented, [and] all *temptation to the commission of the most revolting atrocities removed* [my emphasis].[5]

The concluding comments of the RMS' petition to parliament are emphasised for the light they shed on the controversy surrounding the activities of Burke and Hare and the taint of complicity attached to the name of Robert Knox, extra-mural lecturer in Anatomy in Edinburgh. Students attached to Knox, the most popular lecturer in anatomy in the city, and to rival anatomical lecturers, including Alexander Monro *secundus*, Professor of Anatomy at the University, appeared to be caught up in a feud, which was brought to a head by the scandal over the murders committed by Burke and Hare. On 14 January 1829, at the height of the controversy, an attack was mounted on the library of the Royal Medical Society; the dissertation book was damaged and other papers and catalogues torn. The incident took place after William Burke had been found guilty of murder, and subsequently confessed to involvement in a total of sixteen murders in order to sell the bodies as anatomical subjects, but before his execution and the release of William Hare. The fact that no books were destroyed in the attack on the library suggests that it was the work of student members of the society, but whether they were Knox's supporters or opponents is never declared in the minutes, and the culprits, despite a police investigation, were not traced, although suspicions were aroused:

> It was moved... that the library committee be authorized to take such steps respecting the admission of members to the library during the Evening as may be deemed necessary for the protection of the library...[6]

The vagueness of the minute book references to the incident suggest that a veil was drawn over the controversy, and this method was adopted at times of internal dispute in other medical societies, particularly in regard to breaches of professional ethics.

Debate on the problems of anatomical supply also took place in the Aberdeen Medical Society. Like the RMS, the Aberdeen society had many student members, but it was also the sole medical professional organisation in the city, and this fact gave an additional focus to the considerable controversy which arose when members of the Society became involved with resurrectionist activity. The subject was first broached in 1806, and it was to be raised periodically over the next twenty-five years, as the desire for fresh anatomical specimens was measured against the necessary but highly disreputable and illegal practice of body-snatching, and the effects this activity would have on public attitudes towards the profession. The Aberdeen Society's involvement in resurrectionism was first noted in February 1806,

> On the morning of the 23rd some of the members having procured a subject lodged it in the Society's Hall where in the course of the same day it was unfortunately discovered. At night the body was restored to the Spittal burial ground, from which it had been taken, by some of the members appointed by the President for that purpose one of the Town's Sergeants accompanying them to the grave.[7]

In the event, despite some discussion as to whether the Society should be refused further use of their meeting place (that the body had been lodged in the Society's hall suggests a degree of complicity by the Society as a whole), the members involved were not brought before the court, subject to their paying the cost of the reinterment of their intended subject plus a small fine, and writing a formal letter of apology to the Sheriff.[8]

Again, in 1818, the Society faced the ire of the local authorities in connection with the issue of resurrectionism, the minute book of the 'senior class' (the medical practitioners' section of the Society), noted:

> In consequence of a reference from the council relative to the raising of dead bodies from the Church-yards an extraordinary meeting was [called].... The society ... resolved that the medical men in town should be requested to impress upon the minds of their apprentices the pernicious effects of raising bodies from Church-yards and that the different lecturers

be requested to intimate the same to their students and to discourage the practice as much as lies in their power.[9]

That the issue was still a live one more than a decade later may be seen by a report again in the minute book of the 'senior class', stating that as a result of a wider enquiry into the standard of teaching at King's College, a committee was to be established to write to Doctors Pirie and Ewing, respectively lecturers in Anatomy and Surgery, to dissuade them from encouraging their students to provide anatomical subjects to work on in their classes.[10]

> Dr Dyce reported from the committee appointed at last meeting that they had a meeting with Dr Pirie and that he had declined to enter into any explanation of the manner by which he was to obtain subjects, but he stated that by *an arrangement he had made* [my emphasis] students would not be required to raise subjects and that he would do everything in his power to discourage them from such a practice. Dr Ewing declined to meet the committee...[11]

At the same meeting a letter was read from Ewing resigning from the Society, no doubt feeling that its attempt to regulate the practices of its members was an infringement of his own freedom to run his teaching course as he saw fit. That such activity was going on the year after the notorious enterprise undertaken by Burke and Hare in Edinburgh, which had brought the work of anatomists into public disrepute, suggests that medical professional and student involvement in resurrectionist activity had become deeply ingrained in the practice and teaching of anatomy in this country. Yet it was the local medical society which attempted to regulate professional behaviour in this controversial issue, two years before government legislation on the subject was enacted (although there had been proposals for anatomy legislation in earlier years). The intervention of the Aberdeen Medico-Chirurgical Society notwithstanding, the issue remained a controversial one in the city, as the long-term medical benefits of dissection struggled against the more immediate feeling of the general populace that the medical profession and their hired help by robbing graves were committing a crime against the whole community.[12] In 1832, the anatomy theatre of Andrew Moir, extra-mural lecturer in the subject, was burned down by an enraged crowd estimated at 20,000, after some human remains were uncovered outside it by a dog.[13]

The difficulties faced by surgeons and students in obtaining bodies for dissection in pursuit of the study of anatomy in the early nineteenth century,[14] led in many cases to excesses by these men themselves, as has been shown with reference to the Aberdeen Medical Society, and occasionally to violent opportunism by their suppliers, as in the case of Burke and Hare in Edinburgh in 1828 (although of course, this pair were not 'body-snatchers', but murderers who suffocated their victims and then sold them to Robert Knox). Despite the fact that many practitioners tacitly accepted the necessity of paid procurement of anatomical specimens, Knox was for some years marginalised by his fellow-professionals as a result of his close connection with the activities of Burke and

Hare, although it seems clear that the profession viewed Knox's main crime as the one of being caught.

> Knox, a man of undoubted talent, but notoriously deficient in principle and in heart, was exactly the person to blind himself against suspicion, and fall into blamable carelessness. But it was absurd to charge him with anything worse.[15]

Knox's active intellectual involvement in the Edinburgh Medico-Chirurgical Society and the Royal Society of Edinburgh, which bore fruit in numerous reports of papers in the *Edinburgh Medical and Surgical Journal*,[16] ended abruptly at the end of 1828 and was not resumed until 1836, when papers[17] read before the two societies appeared as articles in the *EMSJ*. Despite this minor recovery, he could not regain his former status among students and his fellow-professionals, and in 1842 Knox eventually left the city in an attempt to resurrect his career briefly in Glasgow, and later in London.[18] No obituary notice appeared in the *Edinburgh Medical Journal* on his death in 1862.[19]

The public perception of the status of the practice of medicine was tainted by the work of resurrectionists and murderers like Burke and Hare, particularly when the indirect benefits of anatomical investigations were measured against the horror felt at the desecration of graves in order to provide specimens for research. The involvement of members of the Royal Medical Society and the Aberdeen Medico-Chirurgical Society in the controversial issue of resurrectionism reflects a wider division within the medical profession, and demonstrates that intellectual development could sometimes rest on sordid foundations. That this illegal practice was eventually resolved by government intervention, in the shape of the passage of the Anatomy Act in August 1832, suggests that the self-regulation of the profession in this matter, as attempted by the Aberdeen Medico-Chirurgical Society, did not provide sufficient control to prevent state intervention in an area of highly contentious medical activity.

PHRENOLOGY

On the evidence of active involvement in medical and related societies, it seems that interest in phrenological science accounted for a large share of Scottish medical practitioners' intellectual activity in the 1820s and 1830s. Nine of the twenty three societies identified in the 1820s and 1830s (see Figure 1.3 in Chapter One) were phrenological societies, which were dominated, if not established, by the local medical profession.[20] It is not the purpose here to enter into the debate regarding the role of the phrenological movement as a popular science,[21] or to suggest that all Scottish medical practitioners at this time were convinced phrenologists, but merely to make the point that until the 1840s phrenology was seen by many in the medical profession nationally as having a legitimate role to play in the expansion of medical knowledge and education. Notable Scottish supporters of phrenology included: William Gregory, Professor of Chemistry at the University of Edinburgh, and Fellow of the Royal Society of Edinburgh; Richard Poole, Proprietor and Superintendent of Middlefield House

Private Lunatic Asylum, Aberdeen, and author of the 'Mental Diseases' section of the *Encyclopaedia Britannia* (7th ed.) among many other articles on mental health; and in Glasgow, William Mackenzie, medical lecturer at Glasgow University, surgeon at Glasgow Eye Infirmary, and Oculist to the Queen in Ordinary in Scotland;[22] and William Weir, co-editor of the *Glasgow Medical Journal*, 1830–32, physician at Glasgow Royal Infirmary, and President of the Glasgow Faculty of Physicians and Surgeons in 1847, a position he held only a year after occupying a short-lived chair of Phrenology at Anderson's College in the city.[23]

It was felt by many of its medical adherents that the study of phrenology could for the first time provide a key to unlock the secrets of the mind, while on a more practical level, analysis of the subject also advanced the study of cranial anatomy. Despite an extensive medico-scientific interest in the subject it remained a contentious topic, and by the early 1840s medical support for phrenology had markedly declined; thereafter, it rapidly moved into the realm of popular culture in which it has firmly remained in the public mind ever since. The subject eventually declined into an area of popular 'pseudo-science', as the early enthusiasm of the medical professional members of the phrenological societies eventually gave way to apathy faced with the limited scope for medico-scientific discussion in a system based on cranial anatomy and categorisation. Phrenology found a new set of supporters more interested in the practical implications of cranial categorisation, and intellectual input into the subject was replaced by the empirical as the 'system' moved from its origins in the anatomy theatre into the showground. The reduction of medical support for phrenology should not, however, mask the fact that for two decades the subject played a role in mainstream medical scientific debate. An early example of this may be taken from the interest displayed in the subject when it was debated before the Royal Medical Society in 1823 by phrenologist Andrew Combe, in his dissertation 'Does Phrenology afford a satisfactory explanation of the moral and intellectual faculties of man?'. A crowd of 400 attended the meeting to hear the dissertation and subsequent discussion which continued for two nights, such was the interest aroused by the topic.[24]

The attempt to locate phrenological science in the mainstream of medical science can be seen in the creation and structure of the Edinburgh Phrenological Society (EPS) in 1820, which displays many similarities to the establishment of 'general interest' medical societies in the same period:

> The objects of the society shall be to hear papers, and discuss questions connected with Phrenology; to hold a correspondence with societies and individuals who may take an interest in the System; and thus to collect and preserve facts and views that may improve and enlarge the boundaries of science.[25]

In common with other medical and scientific societies the EPS consisted of ordinary, corresponding and honorary members. The admission fee was pitched at a high level; two guineas to be followed by a one guinea annual subscription.[26]

Meetings were held fortnightly at 8 p.m. in a session running from November to April. In 1821, the Society reported its early progress in a letter to Franz Joseph Gall 'the "inventor" of phrenology':[27]

> Our Society is not quite so much of a private nature as it formerly was. We have taken apartments in the University [of Edinburgh] where we meet once a fortnight and we have now nearly thirty ordinary members besides corresponding members in London, Dublin, Oxford etc.... There is generally a paper read by some one of the members at each meeting of the Society upon some subject connected with the new System.[28]

It has been suggested by Shapin that the EPS was a group 'on the margins of science' with a membership similarly marginalised from the mainstream of medico-scientific research in the city.

> Phrenology can be fairly precisely located on a social map of the city from the 1810s to the 1830s. Phrenological doctrine (and practice) proved markedly more attractive to 'outsider' intellectuals, and to their audience of superior working-class and petty-bourgeois groups, than it did to establish[ed?] elites. *The University professoriate universally condemned it* [my emphasis]; as did the Established Kirk, the *Edinburgh Reviewers*, and the upper echelons of the legal and medical profession.[29]

Contrary to Shapin's view, and as has already been mentioned, the origins, structure, and membership fees of the EPS bear close comparison to Scottish medical and related scientific societies of the period. The suggestion that the EPS had no links with the scientific investigations of the University of Edinburgh can also be called into question by the fact that the society held its meetings at the University, during its early years at least, as quoted above. Similarly, at least one prominent member of the University's medical faculty had regular contact with the Society. The importance attached by contemporaries to the Edinburgh Phrenological Society's research into cranial anatomy may be measured by the cooperation afforded it by Alexander Monro *tertius*, who had succeeded his father and grandfather as Professor of Anatomy at Edinburgh University. In 1824, a letter was sent thanking Monro for the gift (the third of this nature since 1821) of the cast of the head of Charles MacEwen, a recently executed murderer.[30] Monro's accommodating attitude continued in 1829 when he assented to the Society's request to allow their own sculptor Samuel Josephs access to his anatomy theatre to take a cast of William Burke's head prior to the former anatomical supplier himself becoming a subject for dissection.[31]

It was not only in phrenological societies that medical practitioners discussed the merits of the new 'system'. Two favourable reviews of works on phrenology appeared in the *Glasgow Medical Journal* in 1831,[32] the second of which, on Andrew Combe's *Observations on Mental Derangement* stressed the value of the book for medical practitioners:

> we have only to assure our readers that the present treatise well deserves the attention of medical practitioners, more especially of those who have made mental diseases their particular study.[33]

The Glasgow Medical Society also discussed phrenology on three occasions within the space of a few months in 1825 and 1826, and again in 1837, when local interest in the system had been revived by the re-establishment of the Glasgow Phrenological Society.[34] Only the first of the three papers, delivered by Robert Perry (physician at Glasgow Royal Infirmary) a few months before his election to the Presidency of the Society, was opposed to the practice of phrenology. Perry's essay was a measured assessment based on scientific research, and was not an attempt to ridicule supporters of phrenology in the society.

> From the interest which has been excited in the public mind respecting phrenology, and the fact that it has been embraced by many individuals of considerable research and acknowledged talents, it will at once I think be admitted, that it is a subject entitled to a careful hearing.[35]

Unfortunately, it is not known how Perry's paper was received by the Society since the minutes for the period are extremely brief, noting only the paper's title and the fact of its delivery before the society.[36] Several months after Perry's paper, an essay based on a clinical case history which ended fatally and the subsequent dissection of the brain of the patient in question was read before the Society by the Secretary, in the absence of its author, Alexander Hood, a surgeon from Kilmarnock: 'The appearances on dissection are described, and the connection which these appearances seem to have with the pathology of the brain and the principles of Phrenological Science'.[37] It is important to note that Hood's paper was the continuation of a case history originally outlined in a volume of the *Phrenological Transactions*, and then presented before Glasgow's leading medical society, although again there is no record of the discussion that it provoked.[38]

The third paper delivered on phrenological science before the GMS was given some years later in 1837 by John Maxwell who was at that time President of the Glasgow Phrenological Society. From the tone of his comments it would appear that the ensuing decade and the varying fortunes of the GPS[39] had done little to disprove the scientific basis of the 'system':

> I understand that the discussion of subjects connected with phrenology is not a new thing in this Society. On referring to the table of contents of the volumes containing transactions, I find that two papers connected with that science have been read to its members, some nine or ten years ago. In the interval of time that has elapsed since the reading of these papers, numerous observations in accordance with phrenology have placed themselves in the ranks of its improvers, and much interesting matter has been added to its stock of parts and observations known at that time. We therefore find, as might be expected, the science has already assumed a shape so imposing that the propriety of the question can be no longer doubtful whether its doctrines should be made part of a regular medical education.[40]

The vigour of the reformed Glasgow Phrenological Society is confirmed by an attendance of 191 people at an open meeting of the Society held at the city's Anderson's University in December 1837.[41]

The late 1830s may have been the high point for medical interest in phrenology: after 1840 the minutes of the Edinburgh Phrenological Society show a marked decline in the number of papers read before the Society and an increased emphasis placed on augmenting its collection of head casts and skulls as the medico-scientific elements of Society activity gave way to a more general interest in natural history. The Society was also preoccupied by a claim for a £15,000 legacy bequeathed them by James Robertson, a medical member of the Society who died in France in 1840. The Society spent many years and much of its funds unsuccessfully attempting to free this money by litigation in a saga of Dickensian proportions.[42] The drain on the Society's finances took its toll, and by 1846, the once frequent society meetings were replaced by an annual business meeting at which details of the costs and progress of the legal claim, and a report of new accessions and donations to the museum were the chief concerns.[43] The transition was complete in 1854 when the decision was taken to open up the Phrenological Museum free to members of the public on Saturdays.[44]

In Glasgow, the chair of Phrenology at Anderson's University created in 1845 proved to be something of a nine days' wonder.

> In the year 1845 the managers of Anderson's University in Glasgow resolved to establish a lectureship of Phrenology in that Institution, in which 'The relations of Phrenology to Physiology, Medicine and Education' should be embraced.... Dr William Weir, one of the physicians to the Royal Infirmary of Glasgow, a man of talent, and an able phrenologist was elected to the chair.... These lectures were [however] so little appreciated that a sufficient number of students did not attend to render it expedient to continue them. In consequence, the grant of £50 a-year was withdrawn... Dr Weir resigned, and the lectureship was suppressed.[45]

Only twenty-five students enrolled in the subject in the session 1846–7, and thereafter it was dropped from the University's curriculum.[46] Cooter has made the point that the institution of the lectureship in Phrenology in 1845 was an attempt to revive phrenological science, rather than an indication of its continued relevance to current medico-scientific debate.[47]

The history of the medical profession's involvement with phrenological science aptly demonstrates that an insight into the state of the profession can be gained by the study of the history of medical societies, and that this reflection is not always one of untrammelled progress: the individual members of the medical profession were men of their time and were susceptible to fashionable doctrine in the same way as other citizens. At the same time, close contemporaries acknowledged the medico-scientific benefits of this phase of professional interest. Writing in 1874, Peter Handyside, lecturer in anatomy, and the retiring President of the Edinburgh Medico-Chirurgical Society recognised this:

> One good was effected by this society [the EPS], now I believe, languishing [it ceased existence in 1870], inasmuch as it showed us how little we

knew of the functions of the surface of the brain, though it led us through the admirable instructions of its lecturer, Dr Spurzheim, in the year 1828, to adopt in this School his model of dissecting the fibres of the spinal cord and the enchepalon...[48]

NOTES

1. Creswell (1926), 199.
2. Duncan (1896), 177.
3. In view of my earlier comments on the nature of the society, it is interesting to note that the members of the Royal Medical Society considered themselves as professional medical men, and not students.
4. Royal Medical Society op.cit., minute book, 28 March 1828.
5. Ibid., 8 April 1830.
6. Ibid., 16 January 1829.
7. Aberdeen Medical Society, op.cit., minute book, 28 February 1806.
8. Ibid.
9. Aberdeen Medico-Chirurgical Society op.cit., minute book, 7 December 1818.
10. Aberdeen Medico-Chirurgical Society, op.cit., minute book, 8 July 1830.
11. Ibid., 2 September 1830.
12. For more on this aspect of the history of 'resurrectionism' see Richardson (1987), pp. 90–4 and passim.
13. See Richardson (1987), passim, and Rodger (1893), 231.
14. According to the restrictive anatomy legislation of the period only those executed for a capital offence were released as subjects for dissection by the University Professor of Anatomy ; See Edwards (1977), 120 and passim.
15. Christison (1885, vol. 1), 311.
16. See for example, EMSJ 18 (1822), passim; and for an extensive list of papers delivered by Knox, see Handyside's 'Address to the Medico-Chirurgical Society of Edinburgh', which covers the first fifty years of the history of the Society, EMJ 19/ 2 (1874), passim.
17. EMSJ 46 (1836), pp. 76–89, 89–94, 404–8.
18. For more on the career of Robert Knox, see Lonsdale (1870), and Rae (1964).
19. Rae (1964), 161.
20. There were many other phrenological societies established in Scotland at this time with no prominent medical professional involvement. These are not included in this group.
21. For a survey of the phrenological movement within in the history of scientific debate in this country see Cooter (1984) and (1989); Watson (1836); Shapin, 'Politics of Observation', ch. in Wallis Ed. (Keele, 1979), pp. 138–78; Shapin, 'Phrenological Knowledge' (1975), pp. 219–43; Cantor, 'Phrenology in Early Nineteenth Century Edinburgh' (1975), pp. 195–218; Cantor, 'A Critique of Shapin's Social Interpretation of the Edinburgh Phrenology Debate' (1975), pp. 245–56; Parssinen, 'Popular Science and Society: The Phrenology Movement' (1974), pp. 1–20.
22. Details on the careers of Gregory, Poole, and Mackenzie obtained from the Medical Directory (1861).
23. See Cooter (1984) 298; and GMJ 109 (1928), 76
24. Gray (1952), 134.
25. Printed Laws of the Phrenological Society [of Edinburgh] 1820, Edinburgh University Library Special Collections.
26. This was a relatively high subscription level, and suggests that membership of the EPS was pitched at the leading scientific and medical figures in the community.
27. Cooter (1989), 144.
28. Letter Book of the Edinburgh Phrenological Society 1820–1840, letter from Secretary W. Scott to Gall, 23 January 1821, Edinburgh University Library.
29. Shapin, 'The Politics of Observation' (Keele, 1979) 145.

30. Edinburgh Phrenological Society 1820–40, *op.cit.*, letter book, 15 April 1824.
31. See Edinburgh Phrenological Society *op.cit.*, letter book, 27 January 1829; and EPS minute book, 2 April 1829. Also see Richardson (1987), 32, 'Public dissection of the bodies of executed criminals had a long legal history in Scotland dating from 1506, when James IV granted the Edinburgh Guild of Surgeons and Barbers the bodies of certain executed criminals for dissection...'. The cast of William Burke's head formed part of a renowned collection of skulls and head casts assembled by the EPS many of which may still be seen in the Department of Anatomy museum at the University of Edinburgh.
32. See *GMJ* 4 (1831), pp. 270–9.
33. *Ibid.*, 279.
34. The Glasgow Phrenological Society went through a period of decline in the 1830s. It was first set up in 1829, although interest in phrenology in the city was demonstrated earlier in 1824 at a series of lectures delivered by George Combe. See EPS *op.cit.*, letter book, letter from Secretary, William Scott to a corresponding member of the Society, Charles Caldwell, Lexington, Kentucky, 24 November 1824.
35. Glasgow Medical Society Essays *op.cit.*, vol. 14, Robert Perry 'Remarks on phrenology as connected with the structure of the brain', 5 April 1825.
36. Glasgow Medical Society *op.cit.*, minute book, 5 April 19 1825.
37. Glasgow Medical Society Essays *op.cit.*, Vol. 15, Alexander Hood, 'Continuation of the singular and important case of R. W., narrated at page 235 of the *Phrenological Transactions* and presented to the Glasgow Medical Society', 17 January 1826.
38. Glasgow Medical Society *op.cit.*, minute book 7 February 1826.
39. Cooter (1984), pp. 88–9.
40. Glasgow Medical Society Essays *op.cit.*, Vol. 24 John Maxwell 'On variety in the size and shape of the adult brain and concomitants' 17 January 1837.
41. Anderson's University Popular Evening Classes attendance list 1835–40, 18 December 1837, Strathclyde University Archives.
42. The case was considered in great detail in the minutes for 1841, and subsequently received close attention in the annual reports of the society. See Edinburgh Phrenological Society *op.cit.*, minute book Vol. 2 – 1841–70, *passim*.
43. See EPS *op.cit.*, minute books 1846–70, *passim*.
44. Edinburgh Phrenological Society *op.cit.*, minute book, 11 December 1854.
45. Combe (1850), 481 and note.
46. See Anderson's Institution minute book 1830–64, annual return of students attending the University in session 1846–7, 22 March 1847; and Anderson's Institution Managers' Meeting 3 September 1848, Strathclyde University Archives.
47. Cooter (1984), 96.
48. Handyside, 'Address to the Medico-Chirurgical Society of Edinburgh', (1874) 770.

CHAPTER FIVE

Scottish Medical Societies and the Profession in the Nineteenth and Twentieth Centuries

The main intention of this chapter is to deal with medico-political issues and problems of the profession in the local context. The changing relationship between the local Scottish societies and the expanding British Medical Association is important in this context. A major concern for local medical societies was the development of the auxiliary medical services of midwifery and pharmacy in the course of the later nineteenth and early twentieth centuries. Local medical societies reacted with suspicion. Bearing a distinct similarity to this reaction to the development of auxiliary medical services, is the attitude toward the emergence of female medical practitioners, and their struggle for membership of local Scottish medical societies. The final section of this chapter examines the medico-political issues which came to play an increasingly important role in the daily lives of general practitioners in this period. State involvement in medical care and provision increased, though it was challenged by some local medical societies, who gradually assumed the mantle of local professional pressure groups. In the course of campaigns against growing state regulation of medical provision, local societies on occasion, although not invariably, worked in tandem with the national British Medical Association.

LOCAL COOPERATION AND THE ROLE OF THE BRITISH MEDICAL ASSOCIATION

There was a tendency towards association and geographical union of Scottish medical societies which pre-dated the spread of the British Medical Association branches to Scotland in the 1870s. In 1859, a short-lived Association of Scottish Medical Practitioners was set up in Edinburgh.[1] This Association was formed to promote the enforcement of the 1858 Medical Act, in particular to raise actions for the prosecution of unregistered practitioners. The Association did not last long once it was established that the clauses of the 1858 Act did not extend to such prosecutions,[2] and the next year the Association was described as being in 'a state of suspended animation'.[3]

In the north of Scotland, the Buchan and the Aberdeen Medico-Chirurgical societies, and the Garioch and Northern Medical Association, became affiliated to the North of Scotland Medical Association in 1865, a body set up at the suggestion of the Buchan Medical Society the previous year.

A letter from William Bruce, Secretary of the Buchan Medical Society

[who was later to become Scottish general practitioners' first directly
elected representative on the General Medical Council] dated August 24
1864 was read, to ask, '... if your members would join in an amalgamation
of the different medical societies now existing in the north, to form a
"North of Scotland Medical Association" with meetings yearly in Aberdeen, the present societies, as branches, continuing their independent
existence'.[4]

The NSMA acted as a locus for educational, professional and social interaction
in the region until 1892, when its demise is commented on in the minutes of the
Garioch and Northern Medical Association. 'As the North of Scotland Medical
Association is now an extinct society, no representatives were appointed'.[5]

Interest and support for a medical association covering the north of Scotland
did not necessarily lead to similar enthusiasm for the proposed launching of a
'Scottish Medical Association' in 1874, however. Among the papers of the
Buchan Medical Society there is a collection of documents relating to this
proposed national medical organisation, including a copy of the circular sent by
the committee which had been formed to canvass the opinion of the Scottish
medical societies on the proposal.[6] The letter sent by the Buchan Medical
Society notifying its members of a special meeting to discuss the proposed
national association forms a useful summary, both of the intentions of the
suggested association, and the reasons for the lack of enthusiasm shown in the
north of the country.

> Under the name of the Scottish Medical Association it is proposed to
> unite all existing societies in Scotland, having for its objects the mainte-
> nance of a bond of union among the Members of the Profession in
> Scotland; the elevation of the standard of their attainments, status, and
> emoluments; the defence of their rights and privileges; the cultivation of
> social intercourse; and the advancement of Medical Science.
>
> It is proposed that a General Meeting of the Association be held,
> annually, in each of the four University Seats by rotation.
>
> Practically, the Buchan Medical Society will have to discuss, whether
> they join this National Association, or be content with the General
> Association already in existence, viz., the North of Scotland Medical
> Association.[7]

Given the final paragraph of the above letter, it should come as little surprise
that a limited gathering of the Buchan Medical Society decided by eight votes to
four against offering their support to the proposed Scottish association, particularly bearing in mind the society's formative role in the establishment of the
North of Scotland Medical Association discussed earlier. However, it was not
only north of Scotland medical societies who were unenthusiastic about the idea
of a national association. 'A communication was read from Dr. Strachan[8] of
Dollar about the establishment of a Scottish Medical Association – after some
discussion... the paper was ordered to be left on the table'.[9] From this extract it
would seem the Edinburgh Obstetrical Society did not find great support for the

proposal among its members, and others, including the Forfarshire Medical Association at its annual meeting in Arbroath in 1875, resolved to take no action in response to the circular proposing the setting up of a national medical association.[10]

The largely negative reactions of local medical societies across the country to the proposed Scottish Medical Association may have owed much to the timing of the scheme, mooted at the same time as the BMA was taking its first steps to promote, and in a short period, form local branches of the national Association in Scotland. Certainly, earlier evidence suggests that the union of local societies on a regional and Scotland-wide basis was practicable. Paradoxically, it was an overture from the British Medical Association towards the Scottish Midland and Western Medical Association in 1872 to become a branch of the national Association which led to the proposals for a Scottish Medical Association, as the preferred option of this regional society. The subsequent campaign for an exclusively Scottish association was continued in parallel if not in direct competition to the arrival of local Scottish BMA branches in the 1870s.

The discussion in the SMWMA on becoming a branch of the BMA grew from the fact that, as its name suggests, the Scottish Midland and Western Medical Association had local branches throughout the west and central belt of Scotland, and was, as a society, chiefly concerned with medico-political interests.[11] Yet, despite the preferred option in the ranks of the Scottish Midland and Western of a Scottish Medical Association, there was support for setting up a local BMA branch in the area.[12] There were many individual members of the BMA within the profession in Scotland, including John Mitchell Strachan (Parochial Medical Officer at Dollar), who played a key role in the campaign to set up the Scottish Medical Association, and it was inevitable that a Glasgow and West of Scotland branch of the Association would be established, alongside other regional Scottish branches. Fresh impetus was given to the spread of the BMA in Scotland in 1875 when the Association's annual conference was convened in Edinburgh.[13] The West of Scotland branch, with divisions in Lanark, Renfrew, Stirling, Dumbarton, Ayr, Argyll and Bute, came into being in January 1876.[14] Despite the implied fears of its members, the establishment of the local BMA branch had no adverse effects on the fate or functions of the SMWMA, which continued its strong medico-political activities into the twentieth century, and only in the 1920s did its functions become almost exclusively social.[15]

It is understandable that some societies, such as the SMWMA, viewed the setting up of a local BMA branch in their area as a threat to their independent existence, and mooted a Scottish Medical Association in recognition of the distinct nature of the profession in Scotland. Yet other societies actively encouraged links with the national Association. Local society support for the creation of a local branch of the BMA as in Dundee in 1893,[16] or amalgamation into a regional branch, as in the case of the Perthshire Medical Association in 1888/89,[17] were signs of the vigour of local medical, particularly medico-political, activity in the area.

Local medical societies continued to play an important role in the life of the local profession in the nineteenth and twentieth centuries. This was true despite an apparent fear regarding their long-term prospects engendered by the creation of regional branches of the BMA. Even after the creation of BMA branches, Scottish medical societies maintained an interest in medico-political matters. This was achieved mainly in cooperation, but occasionally in opposition, to the policies of the BMA.

THE CHALLENGE OF THE AUXILIARY MEDICAL PROFESSIONS

It was inevitable that the medical profession in the course of the nineteenth and early twentieth centuries would come into competition with two of what may be termed the 'auxiliary medical services' of pharmacy and midwifery, as the rank and file of the profession emerged from the shadows of corporate dominance by the elite, and began to coordinate pressure group activity on their own behalf through local and national medical societies.

Midwifery

The relationship between the medical profession and midwives has historically been a contentious one[18] with the ascendancy of the often untrained midwife gradually replaced by that of the general practitioner in the late eighteenth century. Despite this, many thousands of women continued to act in this occupation, sometimes in cooperation with the medical profession. As the status of the Scottish medical practitioner rose, so too, was a premium placed on increased levels of training and education, something which the midwife had only limited access to until the twentieth century, and which, in the years after the 1830s, was regularly opposed by the majority of the medical profession who had come to realise the importance of obstetrics in their day-to-day practice and income.

The regulation of women employed as midwives in Scotland was initiated in the eighteenth century in Edinburgh and Glasgow through the Town Council and the Faculty of Physicians and Surgeons respectively.[19] For a short time in the 1820s and early 1830s the Aberdeen Medico-Chirurgical Society revived the notion of instruction for local midwives. In taking on an active role in the regulation and instruction of the medical community, the Society proved to be an exception among the organised medical profession, not simply in these years, but throughout the nineteenth and into the twentieth century.

> It was suggested by Dr Torry that the appointment of a committee to examine and grant certificates to midwives, would tend much to increase the respectability of that class of persons and give the public additional confidence in their skill.[20]

Prospective candidates for examination before the Society were to produce: '1. A certificate of the moral character from the clergyman of the congregation she belongs to. [And, more important], 2. A certificate of having attended one or more courses of lectures in midwifery'.[21] The examination itself covered the anatomy and dimensions of the pelvis and child; the management of labour; and knowledge of after-treatment and related diseases. This scheme lasted for five years between 1827-31, and although reasons for its demise are unclear, acts as a testament to the influence of the Medico-Chirurgical Society within the community. The final report of the scheme in 1831 stated that seventeen midwives had been granted certificates in that year alone, five from the city, and a further twelve from outlying country parishes, where there would presumably be more pressing need for their services.[22]

The need for training and registration of local midwives was not recognised more than sixty years later in 1895 when the progress of the latest in a series of unsuccessful Midwives' Registration Bills then before Parliament was the topic of discussion for the Edinburgh Obstetrical Society. Although this proposal was not intended to cover Scotland, it provoked much heated debate and overwhelming opposition among the ranks of the Society, who viewed any legislation intended to regularise the conduct and enhance the status of midwives as an attempt to undermine their livelihood. In one of the numerous debates on the issue within the Society during 1895, the general tenor of the medical practitioners' opposition to the registration of midwives may be assessed.

> Dr Berry Hart's position briefly was that, keeping in mind the unlikelihood of an effective training for some time, we were face to face with the danger of launching a large number of unqualified women on the public.... Dr. Connel (Peebles) said he preferred the registration of midwifery nurses rather than midwives, though he felt the difficulties. Thirty years ago a sensible neighbour was usually called in, but in his district the doctor was now almost always sent for. This, he believed, was because knowledge had permeated into the minds of the public. If midwives were to be registered, why not also bonesetters?[23]

The Edinburgh Obstetrical Society's opposition to the Bill was in keeping with the prevailing hostile opinion of rank and file medical practitioners, who opposed any attempt to register midwives as a potential threat to their livelihood by the creation of a qualified auxiliary service in direct competition to the medical profession, albeit confined to a single branch of the practice of medicine. Such determined opposition contributed to the delay until 1902 in the enactment of legislation certifying midwives, and the measure when it did come was limited to England and Wales. Certainly the immediate reason for not including Scotland (and Ireland) in the original Bill referred to when it reached the report stage in the House of Commons, would not provide sufficient reason for a twelve year delay in extending the registration scheme for midwives to Scotland.

> Mr. Heywood Johnstone said... with regard to Scotland there did not exist at present any machinery which they could invoke to put the Bill into operation, and a large number of provisions and Amendments would require to be introduced to make the Bill apply to Scotland.[24]

The extension of the Midwives Act to Scotland did not take place until 1915, and when it did come it was supported by the medical profession for personal reasons. Speaking in 1912, the retiring President of the Edinburgh Obstetrical Society laid emphasis on '... the necessity of a Scottish Midwives Bill. It was a necessary antidote, so far as the welfare of women and infants was concerned to the maternity provisions of the Insurance Act'.[25] The occasion for the passage of the 1915 Midwives (Scotland) Act was in part the unprecedented pressure placed on the medical profession during the war as many practitioners enlisted for overseas service. The additional workload this situation created for those remaining at home (and supported by the fact that many Scottish medical societies were held in abeyance for the duration of the war)[26] made for the very speedy passage of legislation to allow for the practice of duly qualified midwives in Scotland. Such provision was now deemed a necessity to ease the pressure on those remaining hard-pressed practitioners who had not signed on for war service. This was made clear in the second reading of the Midwives (Scotland) Bill which was introduced by T. McKinnon-Wood, the Secretary of State for Scotland,

> A great many doctors have gone to the front, leaving rural districts inadequately provided with medical practitioners; so that competent mid-wives are absolutely necessary throughout Scotland.... The Scottish mid-wife is not able to obtain a formal qualification except in England. When she returns to Scotland she is not under the same control as the English midwife is. Altogether, I think, ... [there is a] case for treating this as a matter of urgency ...[27]

The remarkably rapid enactment of the later Bill owed more to the overstretched resources of the Scottish medical profession, rather than to a feeling that the profession of midwifery was long overdue this measure of recognition for its position in the scheme of the nation's health care.

Pharmacy

The activity of the Edinburgh Obstetrical Society noted above, was by no means an isolated instance of the Scottish medical profession's opposition to proposed government legislation on related professions considered to be undermining its status. The level of opposition among the Scottish rank and file practitioners to the professionalisation of midwives was even more intense in regard to the development of the profession of pharmacy in the later part of the nineteenth century, and most vehemently in the early twentieth century. Once again, the roots of the medical profession's opposition dated back as far as the seventeenth century. In Scotland, the tendency towards education in both surgery and pharmacy began as early as the mid seventeenth century,[28] and the development of a tradition of training in both areas was continued through the period of dominance by the Scottish medical schools at Edinburgh and Glasgow Universities, largely remaining unchallenged until the emergence of the dispensing chemist provided an alternative source of prescribed medicines for the wider population.[29]

Many general practitioners in Scotland continued to dispense medicines throughout the nineteenth century as part of their daily practice and this additional source of earnings was for poorer practitioners an integral part of their income. Such practice had by no means disappeared by the twentieth century, although 'shop-keeping' general practitioners had been frowned upon by the upper echelons of the profession for most of the preceding century in terms of the adverse effect such retail practice had on the status of the profession. Whereas the disputes between the pharmacy profession and the medical profession in the first instance, and between the rank and file and the elite of the medical profession in the second, were to reach their most extreme stage in the early part of the twentieth century, a similar set of conflicts emerged in the wake of the passage of the Pharmacy Act in 1868.[30] Many practitioners in the west of Scotland in particular felt that the rights of qualified medical practitioners to dispense restricted drugs and poisons was put under threat by the inclusion of clauses in the Act limiting the sale of such articles by the medical profession to practitioners who had obtained the necessary qualifications from the Incorporated Society of Apothecaries. This seemed to be a threat to poorer practitioners who conducted retail dispensaries to augment their low incomes from private practice. It also threatened the direct income from private practice of this same class of practitioners. By raising the standard of the profession of pharmacy in the public perception, with the outlawing of unqualified dispensers, further encouragement would be given to those of limited means to consult their local chemist or pharmacist for advice rather than paying a doctor's fee. The implications of this piece of legislation for the incomes of medical practitioners' were, therefore, great, particularly when it is alleged that, '... before 1913 around 90% of all dispensing took place in doctors' surgeries...'.[31]

In practice, the follow-up 1869 Pharmacy Act allowed qualified medical practitioners, but not their unqualified assistants, to dispense poisons, who were, however, by necessity, left to tend to the doctor's 'open shop' dispensary for most of the day. This latter point became important in 1900 when the General Medical Council (in the wake of a great surge of prosecutions by the Royal Pharmaceutical Society of Great Britain of medical practitioners for employing unqualified dispensing assistants), charged a number of west of Scotland practitioners with serious professional misconduct for allowing their unqualified assistants to dispense poisons under their names. The immediate result of the passage of the 1868 Pharmacy Act, however, was the combination of three of the Glasgow medical societies, with the Glasgow Southern Medical Society in the vanguard, to coordinate the protest among the city's medical practitioners to its implied threat to their livelihood.

> A conversation on the Pharmacy Act was held after Mr Forrest's reading of the bill with comments. He then proposed that the Act's contents be brought before the Faculty of Physicians and Surgeons and especially those Clauses which seem to interfere with the existing privileges of the licentiates of that body.[32]

The Council of the Glasgow Faculty of Physicians and Surgeons in response to this overture, agreed to send a memorial to the Lord Advocate on the issue, but the Southern Medical Society also decided to establish a committee to continue the local protest activity against the implementation of the Pharmacy Act as it related to the medical profession. Members of two other local societies, the Glasgow and West of Scotland Medical Association and the Glasgow Faculty of Medicine, were also invited to participate on the committee. The latter society had been established to provide poorer Glasgow practitioners with an alternative to the elitist Faculty of Physicians and Surgeons, whose Fellowship was restricted by the high cost of enrolment to the wealthier section of Glasgow medical men.

Perhaps due to the feeling that the Faculty of Physicians and Surgeons would not be supportive on an issue which was of concern chiefly to the rank and file of the local profession, the representative committee of the three Glasgow societies submitted its own memorial to Sir James Moncrieff, Lord Advocate for Scotland.

> The memorialists... respectfully beseech and request your Lordship to take such steps for having said [Pharmacy] act amended, so that it may not... interfere with them in the discharge of their duties; and that the memorialists may be continued in the exercise of the privilege to compound and dispense medicines as hitherto enjoyed by them; and until said act is so amended the memorialists request that your Lordship will not allow any proceedings to be instituted against them should they in the discharge of their duty be obliged to perform any act which may be interpreted as a contravention of the statute.[33]

The passage of the Pharmacy Acts of 1868 and 1869 did little in the short-term to end the practice among rank and file practitioners of keeping 'open shop', as the dispensing and retail of drugs and poisons from the practitioners' own premises was referred to at the time. The continuation of this activity also perpetuated the differentiation in status within the profession in the west of Scotland, as described in the Presidential Address to the Glasgow Southern Medical Society by Robert Forrest senior a local general practitioner in 1872.

> He then referred to the keeping of drug shops by medical men and shewed very satisfactorily that in a city like Glasgow with so many poor, these were indispensable, moreover he contended that as many young medical men when beginning practice were destitute of pecuniary means, it was quite legitimate in them [sic] to make an open dispensary a kind of 'crutch' to assist in gaining an honest living....[Even though] the Faculty of Physicians and Surgeons exclude shop keeping Doctors from their fellowship...[34]

The importance of the Glasgow and west of Scotland practitioners' protest against the clauses of the Pharmacy Act of 1868 is of wider significance than it may at first appear. It reveals a status-related division within the ranks of the medical profession in Scotland, less than a decade after the passage of the

Medical Act of 1858 which, it had been hoped by its advocates, would be a major turning point towards the unification and increasing status of the profession as a whole. The situation changed little in the ensuing thirty two years. The controversy which arose over the employment of unqualified dispensers by medical practitioners in the west of Scotland in 1900–1 demonstrated that the rank and file of the profession faced a struggle against their own governing hierarchy in a way which echoed the clashes in the previous century between physicians and surgeons and their respective governing corporations. This time the governing authority was the General Medical Council, created by the Medical Act of 1858, and the west of Scotland practitioners' ire was directed as much against the GMC, as against the vested interests of the Pharmaceutical Society of Great Britain.

Between 1897 and 1900 the Pharmaceutical Society had instituted 46 prosecutions against medical practitioners in Great Britain for the employment of unqualified dispensers: all of these were against practitioners in the west of Scotland.[35] The court proceedings had little practical effect, as they provoked a sympathetic reaction for the prosecuted from many colleagues. For example, one of those prosecuted in these years, Hugh Arthur, was a member of the Scottish Midland and Western Medical Association, and his case led to a vote of sympathy from the Association.

> It was moved ... and carried unanimously that the sympathy of the meeting be given to Dr Arthur on account of the wrong and annoyance to which he has been subjected on account of the prosecution of his shop assistants.[36]

The Association also decided to refer the matter of the prosecution of unqualified dispensing assistants to the Parliamentary Bills Committee of the BMA. The Committee however, could not offer any support to the position of the shop-keeping practitioners in the west of Scotland, giving as its reason '... it is the duty of the British Medical Association to support the policy of the Pharmacy Acts'.[37] The lack of support from the local BMA branch on this matter of professional and medico-political interest is of consequence given the discussion at the beginning of this chapter regarding the continued role of local medical societies in medical politics in the years after the advent of BMA branches to Scotland.

At the time of his prosecution, Hugh Arthur had been in practice for twenty-five years, was Police Surgeon and Medical Officer of Health for Airdrie Burgh, and physician at Airdrie Fever Hospital, as well as a local parish medical officer and a Public Vaccinator. He was also a member of the BMA and the Medico-Chirurgical Society of Glasgow. His position was not one of a poorly-paid struggling general practitioner, seeking to augment his limited income by dispensing as well as prescribing medicines. While his career may have been the exception which proves the rule, it also suggests that the keeping of 'open shops' for direct dispensing to patients was not simply pursued by recently-qualified practitioners or those in unremunerative private practice, but was an accepted part of private practice in the west of Scotland at this time, hence the unanimous support for him in the ranks of the SMWMA.

With the failure of the mass prosecutions of 1897–1900 to bring any effective implementation of the Pharmacy Acts, the Pharmaceutical Society's lawyers proceeded to take a test case before the General Medical Council in order to attempt to force general practitioners to comply with the relevant Clauses of the Pharmacy Act of 1868. At a hearing of the GMC in London on December 3 1900, the legal advisers of the Pharmaceutical Society:

> referred to the custom prevailing in Scotland of medical practitioners owning chemist and druggist shops, with surgery attached, and pointed out that it was the custom of the medical practitioner to attend a shop for two hours or so and leave the place for the rest of the day in the entire charge of an assistant who was not qualified under the Pharmacy acts of 1852 and 1868. The Pharmaceutical Society regarded this custom as not only contributing a serious danger to the public but as really the 'covering' of unqualified persons so as to enable them to practise [pharmacy].[38]

The irony of a qualified medical practitioner being charged with 'covering' an unqualified assistant cannot be lost, given the fact that so much of the medical profession's political pressure had been directed against just such abuses in the practice of medicine for most of the previous century, yet in the extensive reporting on this issue in the medical press, and as it is discussed in the minutes of the local medical societies, this point is never raised.

The case brought before the GMC was that of John Martin Thomson, a general practitioner in Clarkston, near Airdrie in Lanarkshire, who had been prosecuted on three occasions for employing unqualified dispensers in his shop. The third incident involved the sale of laudanum to a small child whose mother had used the drug to commit suicide. Given the weight of evidence, the GMC found the case against Thomson upheld, but held off from reaching a decision on whether he was guilty of 'infamous conduct', (for which he could be struck off the Medical Register), until the following June. The possible repercussions of this guilty finding by the GMC did not take long to permeate the ranks of the profession in the west of Scotland.

> Sixty four members of the Glasgow Medical profession met in the [Southern Medical] Society's premises to discuss opposition to the recent General Medical Council decision regarding the Sale of Drugs and Poisons by Unqualified Drug Assistants, where it was decided that the body should meet not as the Glasgow Southern Medical Society, but as the 'Practitioners of the West of Scotland'.[39]

Six days later forty five practitioners attended a further meeting which was addressed by William Bruce, the Scottish medical profession's sole directly-elected representative on the thirty one man General Medical Council. '[William Bruce] ... greatly relieved the membership of the general practitioners present by stating that the General Medical Council would never condemn the keeping of open shops'.[40] It was decided to draw up a memorial to the GMC on this issue to be presented in person by a delegation sent from the area, and further, to petition Parliament in an attempt to increase the direct representation of general practitioners on the Medical Council.[41]

It is apparent from these decisions that the case of John Thomson was of importance solely for its symbolic value. For the Pharmaceutical Society his was a test case brought about in order to attempt to enforce the working of the Pharmacy Acts for the benefit of that profession, while for the general practitioners in the west of Scotland the Thomson decision was seen as a blow struck by the supreme governing authority of the medical profession against the ordinary practitioner's freedom to earn a living as best as he or she could. It was regarded by the local profession as a demonstration of the GMC's lack of appreciation of the realities of the day-to-day work of general practitioners. The *Pharmaceutical Journal*, the mouthpiece of the Pharmaceutical Society of Great Britain, understandably took a different view of the GMC's action.

> At last there is a prospect of bringing home to the real offenders what the General Medical Council calls 'a very grave offence', which has been for years a great personal scandal and a serious public danger over a wide area in the West of Scotland. Owing to the persistent and openly defiant action of certain medical practitioners the Pharmaceutical Society has been put to much apparently futile expense, and sheriffs have been subjected to the farce of issuing decrees which could not be enforced. The carefully considered, unmistakeable, and weighty judgement of the General Medical Council has effectually terminated the last hope or shadow of excuse for continuing a practice which is not only a reproach to an honourable profession, but one detrimental to the true interests and progress of both medicine and pharmacy.[42]

The unsurprising support for the GMC's decision found in the pages of the *Pharmaceutical Journal* was echoed in the national medical press at the time, although for reasons altogether different.

> We have no wish to be hard on Dr Thomson. In keeping a shop for the sale of drugs and poisons over the counter, in trade fashion, and without prescribing, he only did what many others of his profession do in his division of the Kingdom. The custom is an old one belonging to more primitive days, and even now in lonely parts it may be capable of some justification. But in general, and at this time of day, it is not one consistent with the welfare of the public or the dignity of the profession, therefore, it must be altered.[43]

The *Lancet*'s sentiment was shared by the *British Medical Journal*,

> That the members of the profession who are affected by the recent decision of the General Medical Council feel somewhat aggrieved is natural.... Although the abolition of the doctor's shop and his unqualified assistant would mean a sacrifice to many in the West of Scotland, it may be nonetheless a desirable result of the present agitation, and would most likely not only benefit the public, but improve the status of the medical practitioner.[44]

It would seem that in the face of such opposition the 'Practitioners of the West of Scotland' had little hope of ultimate success in their rearguard defence of the right to keep 'open shops'. This did not, however, prevent the formation in 1901 of a conjoint committee, consisting of representatives from the Glasgow Southern and Eastern Medical Societies, supported by delegates from the Glasgow and West of Scotland branch of the British Medical Association. The local BMA presence is in contrast to the lack of support given on this issue in 1897. The main objective of this committee was to secure a meeting of its representative deputation with the General Medical Council in June 1901, before the Council reached a decision on the Thomson hearing, to plead their case and to present a petition to the Council signed by 400 medical practitioners from the west of Scotland. This aim was not achieved, as the GMC decided it could not receive a deputation on a case which was *sub judice*. 'June 4th. Early this morning Dr Bruce called at the Hotel and had a prolonged interview with the Members of the Deputation. Regretfully he stated that it was most unlikely that the Deputation would be received'.[45] In the case of John Thomson the GMC decided to take no further action, having restated before him the seriousness with which they viewed his offence. In reaching this decision, the GMC were impressed by the fact that in the intervening six months since his last appearance, Thomson had employed a qualified dispenser to take charge of his shop when he was out on call.[46] It is also possible that the Council was influenced by Thomson's assertion that he was in no way involved in the organised protest against the original decision of the GMC. In fact, according to his *Medical Directory* entries, which cover a period of almost forty years, John Martin Thomson was never a member of any medical society, apart from a brief membership of the BMA in 1923/24.[47]

The matter did not end with the GMC's decision not to remove Thomson from the Medical Register. The repercussions were to be felt in the campaign to elect the Scottish direct representative on the General Medical Council later that year, and also on the hearing of the cases of a further seven medical practitioners from the west of Scotland for employing unqualified dispensary assistants. These cases, which were heard before the GMC in a group, were the result of prosecutions obtained by the Pharmaceutical Society in the wake of the Medical Council's decision in the Thomson case. All seven were found guilty of having committed grave offences against the profession by their conduct. This judgement amounted to a final warning by the GMC, not simply to the practitioners involved, but to the whole of the profession in the west of Scotland, against the employment of unqualified dispensary assistants. To reinforce their decision, the GMC ordered that a warning notice to the profession in the area be published in the local Scottish press.

> the Council hereby gives notice that any registered practitioner who is proved to have so offended is liable to be judged guilty of 'infamous conduct in a professional respect' and to have his name erased from the *Medical Register* under the 29th section of the Medical Act 1858.[48]

The response of the Southern Medical Society (the Conjoint Committee apparently did not last beyond November 1901), was swift, and to a large extent, predictable, 'It is our duty... to protest strongly against the action of the Council in so humiliating men of staunch integrity and of holding up the profession in this part of the country to public ridicule and scorn'.[49] By the time of this meeting the practitioners in the west of Scotland had been dealt a further blow with the defeat of their candidate in the poll to elect a Scottish representative for the Medical Council. Charles Robertson, a general practitioner in the south side of Glasgow came in a poor third[50] to William Bruce who had held the post as directly elected Scottish representative since its inception in 1886. William Bruce had, as has been mentioned earlier, shown some sympathy for the campaign to protect the keeping of 'open shops' by the west of Scotland medical practitioners, and had also supported the calls for the increase of direct representation for the profession on the GMC. Yet Robertson was also defeated in the poll by Norman Walker (assistant physician in the Skin Department of Edinburgh Royal Infirmary), who had declared himself in favour of the GMC's actions against those who maintained retail dispensing outlets in the west of Scotland.[51] His attitude obviously derived more from his belief in the detrimental effects the keeping of 'open shops' had on the profession as a whole, rather than on any geographical bias against practitioners in the west of the country.

The discussion has referred chiefly to the west of Scotland, and it does seem clear that the keeping of 'open shops' by Scottish medical practitioners was geographically limited in the main, to this area of the country.

> Taking the eight largest towns of Scotland, Glasgow, Edinburgh, Dundee, Leith, Aberdeen, Greenock, Paisley, and Perth – we would venture on personal knowledge to say that there are not in them and outside Glasgow, Greenock, and Paisley ten drug shops kept by doctors.[52]

This assessment of course, may have been coloured by self-interest, the pharmaceutical profession seeking to minimise the practice of dispensing by medical men. Evidence for such a conclusion emerges in a further report from the same journal whose comments were noted above, which revealed only three months later, that there were known to be fifteen Aberdeen doctors keeping 'open shops'.[53] It is worth mentioning that both of these reports appeared in 1902, one year after the GMC had issued the warning regarding the employment of unqualified assistants by medical practitioners. It is reasonable to assume that the practice was continuing, since it is unlikely that the many practitioners who continued to retail drugs and poisons would all have taken on qualified drug dispensers, in the face of the additional expense this would involve, and also bearing in mind the questionable availability of such numbers of duly-qualified dispensers. The continued dispensing practices of medical men were in fact, commented on in the *Lancet* in 1905, the general tenor of the discussion bearing a more pragmatic viewpoint than that evidenced by the journal during the struggle between the west of Scotland practitioners and the GMC four years earlier.

There have been many suggestions to make it unprofessional for medical men, save in emergencies, to dispense medicines, and quite recently one of the most important branches of the British Medical Association was asked to pass a proposal, to which effect was later to be given in a Parliamentary Bill, that medical men should cease to dispense. The meeting would have nothing to do with the motion because practical members of the association were alive to the actual conditions obtaining in practice.[54]

This state of affairs continued beyond the passage of the more stringent Poisons and Pharmacy Act of 1908 which demanded that a qualified pharmacist be employed at every retail drug store. The 1908 Act was principally aimed at the emerging chain drug stores such as Jesse Boot's,[55] but would also have had an impact on the shop-keeping general practitioner. It seems clear however, that such legislation could never be strictly enforced as regards the dispensaries of medical practitioners. Indeed, although prescribing and dispensing were finally legislatively separated by the National Insurance Act of 1911,[56] provision was made for local insurance committees to make special arrangements for doctors to dispense in rural areas which had no chemist in the locality. More important was the inclusion in the nine shillings per patient per year capitation fee offered by the government to those members of the medical profession who agreed to join the panel practice scheme of the National Insurance Act in 1911, of eighteen pence for those doctors who supplied drugs to their patients.[57] This should not be taken to imply that all doctors maintained retail outlets, but nevertheless it is clear that some practitioners continued to do so. Even after the panel practice system had been in place for some time, it was still not unknown for Glasgow medical practitioners in certain areas to augment their income by the retail of drugs, in spite of all that had been said from as early as 1868 (from outside the profession and within), regarding the adverse effect such retail trading had on the status of the practice of medicine in general. This is revealed in the autobiography of a local general practitioner, George Gladstone Robertson, *Gorbals Doctor*, in which, referring to the year 1918 when he was still a student, he states:

> I approached my Uncle George [then in general practice in the Gorbals] and asked if I could help him in any way. Without much hesitation he agreed to give me work dispensing medicines, book-keeping and dressing wounds. For this I would be paid two shillings and sixpence per surgery attendance.[58]

The cooperation which was demonstrated among some of the Glasgow medical societies in 1868, and again, in 1900–1, this time also supported by the local branch of the BMA, is not echoed in the minutes of other societies outside the west of Scotland, which made no mention of the issue of the keeping of 'open shops' by Scottish medical practitioners which so dominated the discussions of the Glasgow Southern Medical Society, and also occupied many pages of the national medical press in the early years of this century. Such an omission is surprising, but perhaps indicates that medical societies across Scotland, despite the universal aim of upholding 'professional interests', were as divided on this issue, and its implications for the status of the local practitioner, as was the profession as a whole.

MEDICAL SOCIETIES AND THE ADMISSION OF FEMALE PRACTITIONERS

Thus far Scottish medical societies' activities in the nineteenth and early twentieth centuries have been examined chiefly in relation to their relationship with the British Medical Association, and in regard to the vocal opposition of rank and file practitioners to the professionalisation of midwifery and pharmacy. Also in this period, medical societies provide a unique insight into an area of major professional evolution in the course of the later nineteenth and early twentieth centuries: the emergence of female practitioners.

The impact of the gradually increasing numbers of qualified medical women on the Scottish medical societies at the end of the nineteenth and the beginning of the twentieth century reflects that of their entry into the profession as a whole; prospective female society members were limited in number and encountered a great deal of opposition to their applications. Female medical practitioners in Scotland accounted for 4 per cent of the total number of practitioners in 1911.[59] Yet, as Mary Roth Walsh has argued, for female practitioners medical societies were even more a necessary part of the professionalisation process than for their male counter-parts:

> Medical schools, and societies especially, presented major hurdles.... Nevertheless, women practitioners needed the advantages of professionalization more than men. Female physicians, already suspect because of their sex, required corroboration of their expertise to meet a disbelieving public.[60]

The general hostile response met by female practitioners entering the profession bears similarities to that given to the emergence of the 'auxiliary' medical professions of pharmacy and midwifery, discussed earlier; in both cases the fear of the (male) rank and file of the profession of a threat to their status and income dictated the reaction.

In some Scottish societies there is no record of the subject of the admission of female practitioners being discussed, let alone their becoming members of these organisations. This is particularly true of bodies which met only once a year, such as the Garioch and Northern Medical Association and the Buchan Medical Society. Great store was set by such societies on social functions. In other Scottish medical societies this appears to have played a part in the exclusion of women from membership of what was seen on such occasions as a male dining club, although there were other, less straightforward methods of opposition presented by some male members of medical societies when the question of the admission of female practitioners was raised.

The earliest identified admission of female practitioners to Scottish medical societies took place in 1893. In that year, two female practitioners were admitted to the Glasgow Obstetrical and Gynaecological Society, and the society had eight women members by 1900.[61] Female medical practitioners were also admitted into the Forfarshire Medical Association in 1893. On receipt of a letter from two Dundee general practitioners, Emily Charlotte Thomson (former anatomy demonstrator at the School of Medicine for Women, Edinburgh) and Alice Moorhead (former House Physician at Leith Hospital), requesting to join the Association, the question of the admission of women was opened for debate.

> Dr Lawrence, Montrose, said that... he was of [the] opinion that the presence of ladies at meetings of the Association had certain practical disadvantages, chiefly in the way of limiting freedom of discussion, and he thought that the question should, in the meantime at least, be postponed....
>
> Dr Buist failed to recognize the supposed disadvantages of having ladies present at the ordinary meetings of the Association, and moved that they be frankly admitted to membership.[62]

The motion by Robert Cochrane Buist, Assistant Obstetrician and Gynaecologist at Dundee Royal Infirmary, later Lecturer in Clinical Midwifery and Gynaecology at University College, Dundee, to admit women, was carried by a substantial margin.[63]

The question of the admission of women was raised at the Edinburgh Obstetrical Society in late 1900 in a letter to the Society from Jessie MacGregor, an Edinburgh-based general practitioner, who had previously worked as a resident medical officer at the City's Hospital for Women and Children.

> The Secretary read a letter from Dr Jessie MacGregor to ask if the Society would be willing to elect women to its fellowship. Professor Simpson proposed and Dr Aitchison Robertson seconded that women should now be admitted. This motion to come up for discussion and ballot at the next meeting.[64]

The motion was passed unopposed, and at the next meeting Jessie MacGregor and Hilda M. MacFarlane, also an Edinburgh graduate, who was employed at Northumberland County Asylum, were both admitted as fellows of the Society.[65]

In 1903, the members of Glasgow Medico-Chirurgical Society attending their AGM in May of that year, acting on the unanimous advice of the council, voted in favour of allowing female practitioners to join the Society. However, in October 1903 the admission of female members was successfully opposed on procedural grounds by George Stevenson Middleton, physician at Glasgow Royal Infirmary, and a former President of the Society, who argued that the admission of an unnamed female practitioner was invalidated by the fact that only her name and initials appeared on the proposal form, hence members did not know for whom they were voting. This dubious manoeuvre to continue to exclude female practitioners from Glasgow's leading medical society succeeded, and it was not until May 1911 that the motion, 'That women shall be eligible for election as ordinary members on the same terms as presently apply to men' was accepted by the Society, by a margin of sixteen votes to four.[66]

Middleton had less success in his attempts to block the admission of female practitioners to the Glasgow Pathological and Clinical Society in November 1903. His objection to the motion to admit women on the grounds that:

> the usefulness of the Society would be limited by the admission of Lady members. It must be borne in mind that the Society is a Clinical as well as a Pathological one, and that at times the cases of patients are presented to the Society whose complete demonstrations, would, in the presence of Lady members, constitute a real difficulty,[67]

was defeated by twelve votes to seven.

The admission of women to membership of the Aberdeen Medico-Chirurgical Society in 1905, went unremarked at a time when the minute book entries for the Society were brief and formalised, giving no idea of any debate or dissension among the members on the issue.

> The minute of the previous meeting having been read and approved of, Drs Laura Sandeman and Ann Mercer Watson were nominated as members of the Society....
>
> ... After the minutes of the previous meeting had been read and approved of Dr Laura Sandeman and Dr Ann Mercer Watson were balloted for and admitted [as] members of the Society.[68]

There was no such reticence displayed on the matter of the admission of women to the Glasgow Southern Medical Society. The subject was first raised in 1895[69] and a vote was taken on the issue in February 1896. At this meeting six members of the Society supported the direct negative to the motion to admit women, while three others were in favour of it. The remaining four members in attendance remained undecided until one of the opponents of the motion brought the debate to a close.

> Dr Hamilton... deprecated the absence of the senior members of the Society, and some of the changes which had occurred in recent years. The society was one in the first instance for general practitioners. Were the motion to be carried the society would lose its particular attributes.[70]

This call to tradition carried the day, with five members eventually supporting the motion, and eight opposing it.[71] The issue was raised again in 1900 during the course of a revision of the Society's constitution and bye-laws, and was again defeated, this time by eight clear votes.[72] The matter was apparently not raised again until the 1926/27 session when a retired practitioner, Robert Forrest junior, a former House Physician at Glasgow Western Infirmary, spoke in favour of a motion to admit women in terms of the granting of equal rights to women, which was gradually being acknowledged by the profession as a whole, and could be witnessed in the admission of women to most of the other Glasgow medical societies. This motion was directly opposed by the then Secretary of the Society, Osborne Henry Mavor, Assistant Physician at Glasgow Victoria Infirmary, (better known as playwright and misogynist, James Bridie), and once again the call to the 'traditions' of the Society won the day.

> He said that our society had been founded over eighty years ago as a peculiarly male phenomenon and he thought that it still provided for its

members a social atmosphere that the admission of ladies [sic] could not fail to destroy.[73]

Again, the Society rejected the proposed admission of women, although on this occasion the ballot was closer, with the 'traditionalists' view prevailing by a margin two votes in favour of Mavor's negative. Although there were further discussions on the issue in 1928, this was as close as women were to come to admission to the Society until they finally gained entry in 1979.

Perhaps due to the refusal to admit female members to the Society twice in the space of three years, a Glasgow Southern Women's Medical Society was established at some time before March 1928. Knowledge of this body came to light somewhat strangely, due to the fact that the Women's Society began to hold joint meetings with the older body from 22 March 1928. 'This was a notable occasion in the society's history, in that the meeting was a joint one with the Glasgow Women's Southern Medical Society...'[74] These joint meetings were continued for at least three years, after which they are no longer mentioned, perhaps the GSWMS feeling that cooperation with a society which refused to admit them as full participating members was anachronistic.

The first Scottish society set up by and for female practitioners had appeared at the very end of the nineteenth century. From the outset, and by necessity, these organisations contained a large element of professional self-help. The Edinburgh Medical Women's Club (later renamed the Scottish Association of Registered Medical Women in 1906) was established by female graduates of the Edinburgh Extra-Mural Medical School in 1899, among them Jessie MacGregor, mentioned above as one of the first female members of the Edinburgh Obstetrical Society, and her partner in general practice, Elsie Inglis. Members of the club also set up a small private nursing home to provide maternity care for women, which later amalgamated with Bruntsfield Hospital.[75] In 1904, the Glasgow and West of Scotland Association of Registered Medical Women was established, and from the beginning its objects were professional and social, rather than educational: '1. To form a bond of union among the women in practice in Glasgow and the West of Scotland. 2. To look after the interests of medical women generally'.[76]

Both of these local associations became part of the national Medical Women's Federation on its launch in 1917, under the titles of the Scottish Eastern and Western Associations respectively (acting jointly as the Scottish Medical Women's Union for issues of a purely Scottish medical professional nature). They were joined in the Federation in 1927 by the Aberdeen and North of Scotland Association of Medical Women.[77] The activities of the Medical Women's Federation were directed towards achieving professional parity with male practitioners, particularly in terms of equality of employment opportunities and salary, and in this the Federation often worked closely with the British Medical Association, professional integration rather than separation providing the key element to the Federation's activity. The great need for the professional pressure group activities of the MWF can be highlighted by the campaign for equality of opportunity in public medical appointments in Glasgow after 1921. The BMA Medico-Political Committee's minutes for 22 April of that year reported on their joint efforts with the MWF in protest against the proposal (later implemented), by Glasgow Corporation to dismiss four women doctors from public medical appointments as part of a general campaign to dismiss all married women who had husbands working, from the corporation's employ, and to replace them with the single unemployed.[78] The female practitioners in question had been employed as medical officers in the tuberculosis and child welfare departments. The concentrated efforts of the MWF and BMA notwithstanding, the marriage bar on female employees with working husbands continued beyond the period under survey, as revealed in a protest letter directed to Glasgow Corporation by the MWF in July 1947: 'The Medical Women's Federation is deeply concerned to learn that the City of Glasgow continues to enforce a marriage bar on its medical women employees'.[79]

That female medical practitioners were still the subject of discrimination for official medical posts in Glasgow in the period after the Second World War suggests that the work of the MWF and its local Scottish associations remained essential even in the mid-twentieth century, and that the role of the medical society as a medico-political pressure group remained a key one.

THE PROFESSION AND THE STATE IN THE EARLY TWENTIETH CENTURY

The increasing involvement of the state in medical provision in the early years of the twentieth century posed a much more direct set of problems and challenges for the profession as a whole than those discussed in Chapter One in connection with the beginning of medico-political pressure to force government activity in the realm of medical education: the first seemed to be an expression of growing professional awareness, the second was provoked by a fear that hard-fought professional independence was about to be undermined by state involvement in the provision of national medical services. The activities of local medical societies in the period between 1908 and 1913 provide valuable evidence as to the negative reactions of Scottish general practitioners to the introduction of a salaried school medical service, and, perhaps more well known, to the implementation of the National Health Insurance Scheme. A consideration of these activities also reveals the continued importance of the local societies, in an area where the role of the BMA has hitherto been considered as paramount.[80]

School Medical Officer Appointments

The advertisement for part-time medical officers by Glasgow School Board in 1909 created a situation which led to division within the profession in the city, and within the membership of both the Glasgow Southern Medical Society, and the local BMA branch. The majority of the members of both groups opposed such appointments as undermining the independence and level of remuneration of the profession, by removing from private practice to salaried government service at one fell swoop, a whole section of the population, and therefore, placing in the hands of a select few, a fixed income for seeing cases which would normally have been treated on an individual basis by general practitioners. In practice, this argument proved spurious, and the profession's fears of reduction of income, groundless. Most of the children treated as a result of medical inspection at school had formerly been left unattended by medical care in any form, due to a combination of family poverty and general ignorance of their conditions. In other words, the appointment of school medical inspectors provided for a level of general preventive health care hitherto beyond the capabilities of individual general practitioners, however well-intentioned. This is made clear by an early report on the functions of the School Medical Service in Edinburgh quoted in the *Lancet*.

> An account has been published of the scheme of the Edinburgh school board for the medical inspection of school children.... Under the scheme the staff carries out regular visitations of the schools, examination of the pupils, and supervision of cases in which parents are suspect of neglect. The board is proceeding under two statutes – the Education (Scotland) Act, 1908, and the Children Act, 1908.... No powers are given to the board to provide treatment, the duties of the medical officers being to examine the children, report defects to parents, and bring to the notice of the board children suffering from neglect or cruelty at home.... It is stated that already there is a marked improvement in the condition of children, concerning whom reports have been made to the parents, and that considering the home conditions the efforts made to keep the children clean and wholesome in many cases are surprising. The board is now making arrangements to provide food for the underfed children in the schools...[81]

That there was clearly a great demand for the endeavours of a school medical inspectorate can be demonstrated by the fact that the activities of the service were being supported illegally by Scottish local authorities loosely interpreting the conditions of the Education (Scotland) Act of 1908 to enable them to draw upon the rates.[82] The obvious need for a school medical service notwithstanding, there was considerable opposition to the introduction of a salaried school medical inspectorate among the members of the Scottish medical societies, in Glasgow, as has been mentioned, but also in the north of Scotland:

> A discussion took place on the County Council scheme for the examination of school children. The feeling was that the proposed scheme was too expensive... and that after the first [examination] of the schools, the work would swiftly become a sinecure.[83]

Such objections were soon to be succeeded by a considerable outcry against those practitioners who accepted appointments as school medical officers. The Council of the Glasgow Southern Medical Society recommended:

> That the Society records in the minutes its high appreciation of the conduct of those practitioners who, in deference to the opinion of the local profession as expressed at a duly convened meeting of medical men...

withdrew their applications or abstained from applying for posts of part-time officers as advertised by Glasgow School Board; and further 'that members who, notwithstanding the opinion of the meeting referred to, have accepted these positions under the Glasgow School Board, should in the circumstances resign their membership of the Glasgow Southern Medical Society'.[84]

It is clear that the Glasgow and West of Scotland branch of the BMA had acted in a similar fashion from a reference in 1912 to the reinstatement of two former members who had been compelled to resign their membership sometime previously owing to their acceptance of School Board appointments.[85]

The organised opposition to the introduction of a salaried school medical service was in part countered by the creation of an Association of School Medical Officers of Scotland[86] in 1911 to protect the interests of this section of the medical profession. The creation of this Association is an indication that even in the twentieth century the setting up of medical societies could be a sign of division, rather than unity in the profession.

That the introduction of a salaried school medical service remained worthy of comment at a time when the profession was apparently involved in a life and death struggle with the government over the National Health Insurance Scheme, is indicative of how far both of these issues can be regarded as part of a wider campaign of resistance by the majority of the profession to increased government intervention in the area of health care and the regulation of those who provided it.

In 1908, the year before the introduction of a salaried School Medical Service, fear of state intrusion into their professional activities had provoked the Aberdeen Medico-Chirurgical Society to vigorous protest against the Town Council's proposal to adopt the 1907 Notification of Births Act in the locality.[87] Early in 1908, a representative deputation was chosen to present a memorial to the Council which objected not to the objects of the Act, but to the method of its proposed administration,

> namely, by means of gratuitous certificates supplied under penalty by medical men attending births... the injustice to medical men of expecting them to perform another gratuitous service to the State was [stressed].... This vigorous defence of professional rights may be commended to the notice of medical societies everywhere.[88]

National Health Insurance

The 'vigorous defence of professional rights' highlighted by the activities of the Aberdeen Medico-Chirurgical Society in opposition to the implied extra unpaid responsibility placed on the medical profession in the operation of the Notification of Births Act, was soon to be echoed throughout the country as the majority of the profession reacted negatively to the medical provisions section of the National Insurance Scheme. The degree of unanimity with which the British medical profession greeted the introduction of the then Chancellor of the

Exchequer, Lloyd George's, National Health Insurance Bill to parliament on 4 May 1911 was remarkable, and soon led to support being very firmly channelled behind the protest activities of the British Medical Association.

> The committee... [appointed by the Aberdeen Medico-Chirurgical Society to monitor the passage of the Bill] desire in the first place to impress upon the members of the Society the absolute necessity for unanimity and combination on the part of the profession.... In view of the important steps being taken to defend the profession by the British Medical Association the committee feels any independent action by the Society would be inadvisable at this juncture.... The committee would further recommend that each of the members of the Society should sign the circular to be sent out by the British Medical Association, by which he [sic] pledges himself not to enter into any arrangements for the treatment of patients under the Insurance Scheme except under the conditions defined in the policy of the Association.[89]

A special meeting called by the Buchan Medical Society to discuss the Bill echoed the sentiment, 'No one of us will agree to act for any of the friendly societies, without the consent of the members of this Society and according to the policy of the British Medical Association'.[90]

The two major areas on which the BMA protest campaign was focused, namely, the pledge to refuse service in any proposed scheme for National Insurance, and the refusal to carry out contract practice by those practitioners already employed by Friendly Societies (who originally were to be given much of the responsibility for administering the new national scheme), produced dramatic results. Throughout Great Britain 26,000 medical practitioners signed the BMA pledge, and more than 33,000 contract medical appointments were terminated. Such support for their campaign saw the BMA (which was acting in this instance in a manner not unlike that of a trade union for the first time in its history), secure many of its aims in the revision of the National Insurance Bill, (achieving acceptance of four of its six so-called 'Cardinal Points') during negotiations with the government.[91] For most of 1912 the need for a unified front on the part of the profession was recognised and maintained, but towards the end of that year as the date for the implementation of the scheme of medical benefit to be provided through the panel-practice system in January 1913 loomed, divisions began to appear, and local medical society support for the BMA's hardline became equivocal, particularly in view of the BMA leadership's apparent intransigence and unwillingness to continue negotiations with the government in the hope of a last-minute settlement which would allow the profession to work within the scheme.

A special meeting called by the Buchan Medical Society in December 1912 reveals the turmoil within the membership of the local Scottish medical societies.

> The question of breaking our pledge to the British Medical Association and joining the Panel of the National Insurance Bill[sic] was discussed....

All present expressed their opinions on the question but the majority were against breaking our pledge and joining the panel. A vote, however, was not taken till we found by telephone that the [BMA] Branch meeting in Aberdeen, by which we are to be guided, declared by 47 votes to 32 in favour of joining the panel. It was then declared that, being at liberty to join the panel, we should all do so.[92]

A similar decision was almost simultaneously being reached at the Council meeting of the Glasgow and West of Scotland branch of the BMA:

The Branch Council suggests that all members who dissent from the present policy of the Association, whether or not they intend to apply for service upon the panel, should sign the accompanying form and return it at once to the Secretary of the Branch.... 'In view of the altered circumstances I beg to give you formal notice that I herewith withdraw from the undertaking and pledge of the British Medical Association'.[93]

The increasingly ambiguous Scottish support for the actions of the BMA suggested by the two above extracts, can be substantiated by an examination of the local divisional returns of the nationwide ballot the Association conducted on 14 December 1912, which show a distinct national split in levels of support for the last-ditch tactics of the BMA.

The crucial nationwide doctors vote on December 14 showed a remarkable result. When the votes of the individual medical district organisations throughout England, Wales and Scotland were recorded, it showed that in England only two out of 88 BMA divisions favoured the Scheme. In Scotland, however, eight out of sixteen divisions voted for it, and substantial majorities for the Scheme were recorded in Ayrshire and Dundee. Glasgow was only narrowly against the Scheme, but Edinburgh, Perth and the Borders were strongly opposed. The vote thus corresponded to the amount of individual practice carried out by the doctors.[94]

Even the *Edinburgh Medical Journal* which had until the end of 1912 been a redoubtable supporter of the BMA's tactics had to concede that the Association no longer spoke for the majority of the profession on the issue of the National Health Insurance Scheme,

The Association has certainly not proved what was hoped, and, as events showed, the last move was a tactical error. The Association, for the time being, ceased unequivocally to represent the profession, and many of its members absolved themselves from their pledges in consequence.[95]

Having been directed by the actions of the BMA, who in the latter part of 1912 and beginning of 1913, clearly seemed to have lost touch with the opinions of the rank and file of the medical profession, the Scottish medical societies also suffered the same hangover effects as the national association in the wake of the long struggle with the government over the state's role in national health provision, with a drop in membership and attendance at meetings. In the case of the BMA, its membership dropped sharply in the period 1913 to 1918, owing partly to the effects of the War on the profession, but also due to a feeling of disillusionment with the efficacy of professional union in the face of government intervention.[96] The annual report of the Forfarshire Medical Association in 1913 remarked that a fall in the average attendance at Association meetings during the previous session, was due:

> [To] a weariness of the flesh brought about by a plethora of meetings of an entirely different character, during a time of unparalleled anxiety in the profession, the exciting cause being the Insurance Act. As the refreshing fruit has now ripened to maturity, it is to be hoped that the Association will regain next session its normal appetite for scientific dietary.[97]

Similar poor attendances affected the Glasgow Southern Medical Society as the Secretary's annual report in April 1913 made clear,

> Though several of the meetings had been well-attended, notably the social functions, the average attendance especially in the latter part of the session, had been disappointing, so much so that the Council had decided to terminate the session at an earlier date than usual. A reason for the falling off might be found in the disturbing influences of the inception of the Insurance Act...[98]

The 'disturbing influence' of the implementation of the National Health Insurance Act on the profession's self-esteem was not a permanent one, however, as the functioning of the Act proved not to be the great disaster for the profession that had been predicted, and the benefits of panel practice for the standards of health care were becoming evident, aided by the fact that a separate administrative framework for operating the scheme in Scotland (and in Wales) had been established. The belated acceptance by the profession of the great changes wrought in health provision by increased state intervention emerged at a meeting of the Glasgow Southern Medical Society in December 1913 devoted to a review of the first year's operation of the National Insurance Act.

> Fears, which existed before the Act was passed, of unreasonable demands being made by patients on the practitioner had been found in his experience and in that of others, not to have been realised. The effect of the Act on the morale of either patient or doctor was not on the whole, in Dr. Drewer's opinion, for the worse. Malingering was not prevalent and though the sick benefit expended had been very much greater than the Societies had anticipated this was not due to Malingering but to the fact that great numbers could now afford to wait until they were reasonably well before resuming work where formerly they were often compelled by necessity to work before completely well.[99]

While this view did not perhaps take into account some of the difficulties which the working of the scheme were to raise, not the least of which was to be the level of per capita payment for panel medical practitioners, the change in attitude here displayed by the profession in the course of one year, is remarkable.

In the early years of the twentieth century, the opposition of the medical profession, as voiced in the minutes of Scottish medical societies, was focused on the increasing intervention by the government in the actual practice of medicine and the regulation of the levels and nature of the nation's health provision. Such intervention was regarded by the majority of those involved in medical practice as an attempt to reduce their independent status as providers of health care, to the role of government agent; to all intents and purposes little more than the reduction of the profession to that of a medical civil service. In practice, such fears proved in most respects unfounded, although there was an increase in the clerical and supervisory duties of panel practitioners. Yet this was not so far removed from the activities of contract medical appointees to Friendly Societies in the pre-Insurance era. Perhaps the greatest change in regard to the profession as it is reflected in the records of the Scottish medical societies, is a shift away from nineteenth century discussions on the means of protecting and enhancing the status of the profession, towards those on the role of the profession in the twentieth century within the context of the ever-increasing state involvement in medical concerns.

The intention of this chapter has been to examine some of the chief professional and medico-political interests of Scottish medical societies in the later nineteenth and twentieth centuries as representative of the issues dominating the concerns of rank and file medical practitioners in these years. It is no coincidence that much of the discussion has focused on the professions' relationship with the state, at a time when government involvement in national medical provision was presenting a new series of challenges to the profession of medicine.

Other areas tackled in this chapter, namely the rise of the auxiliary medical professions, and the emergence of female practitioners, echoed the profession's struggle to exclude 'irregulars' from the practice of medicine in the early nineteenth century, when the new-found status of the profession was apparently being challenged from rival occupations. The difference in the later period was in the attempt to preserve the status quo rather than a campaign for reform, an indication of the great strides made in the status of medicine as a profession in the intervening years.

The shifting relationship between local medical societies and the British Medical Association was important in the campaign of organised opposition to the government's attempt to impose a scheme of national health insurance on a largely unwilling medical profession between 1911 and 1913. This can be seen first of all in the impressive success of the BMA backed by the local societies in forcing changes in the government proposals, and then in local society disenchantment with the national Association's increasingly hard-line attitude, which helped hasten the eventual acceptance of the reformed government scheme. Even in times of apparent crisis for the profession nationally, such as the final months of the struggle over the National Health Insurance Scheme in 1912, medical societies retained their local dimension and independence.

NOTES

1. See Chapter One, pp. 17–8, for more on this Association.
2. *EMJ* 5 (1859–60), 967.
3. *Ibid.*, 6 (1860–1), 775.
4. Aberdeen Medico-Chirurgical Society *op.cit.*, minute book 3 November 1864.
5. Garioch and Northern Medical Association *op.cit.*, minute book, 24 September 1892.
6. Buchan Medical Society *op.cit.*, printed circular on 'The Scottish Medical Association', dated 6 November 1874.
7. Buchan Medical Society *op.cit.*, printed notice of special meeting, 4 October 1875.
8. John Strachan, a general practitioner in Dollar, Clackmannanshire, was one of the leading figures behind the campaign for a Scottish Medical Association. An office-bearer with both the Scottish Midland and Western Medical Association, and the Clackmannan and Kinross-shire Medical Association, he was also a member of the Harveian, Royal Medical and Edinburgh Medico-Chirurgical Societies.
9. Edinburgh Obstetrical Society *op.cit.*, 9 December 1874.
10. See the report of the 17th annual meeting of the Forfarshire Medical Association in *EMJ* 21/1 (July–December 1875), 170.
11. See Scottish Midland and Western Medical Association *op.cit.*, minute book 1873–1928 *passim.*
12. Scottish Midland and Western Medical Association *op.cit.*, minute book, 13 July, 12 October, 1875; 14 January, 13 October 1876, *passim.*
13. For details of the formation of Scottish regional branches of the British Medical Association and more on the impact of this on local medical societies, see Jenkinson 'Role of the Medical Societies' (1991), pp. 269–272.
14. Little (1932), 50.
15. See Scottish Midland and Western Medical Association *op.cit.*, minute book, 1921–39 *passim.*
16. Jenkinson 'Role of Medical Societies' (1991), 271.
17. *Ibid.*
18. For a useful discussion (although relating predominantly to England) of the relationship between midwives and the medical profession, see Donnison (1977), *passim.*
19. Donnison (1977), pp 22–3.
20. Aberdeen Medico-Chirurgical Society *op.cit.*, minute book, 5 October 1826.
21. *Ibid.*, 5 April 1827.
22. *Ibid.*, 3 November 1831.
23. Edinburgh Obstetrical Society *op.cit.*, minute book, 20 July 1895.
24. *Hansard*, Vol. 109, 6–24 June, 1902, cols., 58–9.
25. *BMJ* pt. 2 (1913), 1103.
26. See for example, Aberdeen Medico-Chirurgical Society *op.cit.*, minute book, 19 November 1914 and Glasgow Southern Medical Society *op.cit.*, minute book, 11 November 1915.
27. *Hansard*, Vol. 76, 22 November–17 December, 1915, cols. 480–1.
28. See Chapter Three, p. 54, for more on this subject.
29. For a useful discussion (although mainly limited to the English context) of the dispensing activities of general practitioners and the emergence of pharmacy as a separate and potentially rival profession, see Loudon (1986), pp. 129–51 *passim.* For more on the history of pharmacy in Britain see Holloway (1991).
30. Holloway (1991), 165, has pointed out that both Scottish corporations which represented surgeons, opposed the earlier Pharmacy Act of 1852, '... under the impression that it would interfere with their right to practise pharmacy : amendments were made to conciliate them'.
31. Stewart, 'Jubilee of the National Insurance Act' (1962), 33–5.
32. Glasgow Southern Medical Society *op.cit.*, minute book, 29 October 1868.
33. *Ibid.*, 3 December 1868.
34. *Ibid.*, 31 October 1872.
35. See Holloway (1991), 283. Holloway's figure is in fact forty-five, the slightly higher figure is taken from contemporary accounts of the prosecution by the Pharmaceutical

Society of John Martin Thomson in December 1900 for employing an unqualified dispenser, for example see *Lancet* 8 December 1900, 1694.

36. Scottish Midland and Western Medical Association, *op.cit.*, minute book, 11 March 1897.
37. *Ibid.*, Quarterly Council meeting, 15 April 1898.
38. *Lancet* 8 December 1900, 1694.
39. Glasgow Southern Medical Society *op.cit.*, minute book, 14 December 1900.
40. *Ibid.*, 20 December 1900.
41. *Ibid.*
42. *Pharmaceutical Journal* 8 December 1900, 648.
43. *Lancet* 5 January 1901, pp. 44–5.
44. *British Medical Journal* 5 January 1901, 50.
45. Conjoint Committee of the Glasgow Southern and Eastern Medical Societies and the Glasgow and West of Scotland Branch of the British Medical Association, minute book, 14 June 1901, Victoria Infirmary Library, Glasgow.
46. *Lancet* 8 June 1901, pp. 1641–2.
47. See *Medical Directory* 1893–1930, *passim*.
48. *British Medical Journal* 7 December 1901, pp. 1699–1700.
49. Glasgow Southern Medical Society, *op.cit.*, minute book, 19 December 1901.
50. See result of the poll, *British Medical Journal* 14 December 1901, 1766.
51. *Lancet* 16 November 1901, pp. 1364–5.
52. *Chemist and Druggist* 15 March 1902, 429.
53. *Ibid.*, 28 June 1902, 902.
54. *Lancet* 1 April 1905, 879.
55. *Hansard* Vol. 197, 24 November–4 December 1908, col. 1715.
56. Holloway (1991), 335.
57. Gilbert (1966), 411.
58. Robertson (1970), 41.
59. Dupree and Crowther, 'Profile of the medical profession in Scotland' *Bulletin of the History of Medicine* 65 (1991), 217.
60. Walsh (1977), 15.
61. See printed membership list in *Transactions of the Glasgow Obstetrical and Gynaecological Society* (1901), pp. xi–xiv. There is no surviving minute book for this period.
62. Annual report of the Forfarshire Medical Association, 29 June 1893, Dundee University Archives.
63. *Ibid.*
64. Edinburgh Obstetrical Society *op.cit.*, council minute book, 12 December 1900.
65. *Ibid.*, 9 January, 13 Febuary, 1901.
66. Medico-Chirurgical Society of Glasgow *op.cit.*, minute book, 5 May 1911, *passim*.
67. Glasgow Pathological and Clinical Society, minute book, 9 November 1903, Library, Royal College of Physicians and Surgeons, Glasgow.
68. Aberdeen Medico-Chirurgical Society *op.cit.*, minute book, 4 May and 2 November 1905.
69. Glasgow Southern Medical Society, *op.cit.*, minute book, 28 November 1985.
70. *Ibid.*, 6 February 1896.
71. *Ibid.*
72. *Ibid.*, 18 January 1900.
73. *Ibid.*, 15 April 1926.
74. *Ibid.*, 22 March 1928.
75. See Papers of the Medical Women's Federation, *op.cit.*, MS History of Bruntsfield Hospital by Joan Rose, May 1947.
76. Session card of the Glasgow and West of Scotland Association of Registered Medical Women 1905–6, among papers of the Medical Women's Federation *op.cit.*
77. Medical Women's Federation *op.cit.*, Council minute book, 12 November 1927.
78. See 'Married women and medical appointments 1919–1954', British Medical Association Medico-Political Committee Minutes, 22 April 1921, among papers of the Medical Women's Federation *op.cit.*
79. Medical Women's Federation *op.cit.*, letter from Medical Women's Federation to Glasgow Corporation 17 July 1947.

80. See for example, Little (1932), 324–32; and Brand (1965), 216–31. Other historians have given some attention to the opinions of those opposed to the BMA's campaign, see Gilbert (1966), 400–15, and Eder (1982), 31–45.
81. *Lancet* 2 November 1910, 1518.
82. McLachlan (1987), pp. 55–6.
83. Buchan Medical Society *op.cit.*, minute book, 25 September 1909.
84. Glasgow Southern Medical Society *op.cit.*, minute book, 27 December 1909.
85. Glasgow and West of Scotland Branch of the British Medical Association, minute book 1910–18, 25 October 1912, Victoria Infirmary Library, Glasgow.
86. See entry 9 in Part Two of this book for more on the Association of School Medical Officers for Scotland.
87. Aberdeen Medico-Chirurgical Society *op.cit.*, minute book, 9 January 1908.
88. *Lancet* 8 February 1908, 461.
89. Aberdeen Medico-Chirurgical Society *op.cit.*, minute book, 6 June 1911.
90. Buchan Medical Society *op.cit.*, minute book, 24 June 1911.
91. For a discussion of the BMA's campaign against the National Health Insurance Scheme see Little (1932), pp. 324–8; and Brand (1965), pp. 224–5.
92. Buchan Medical Society *op.cit.*, minute book, 28 December 1912.
93. BMA, Glasgow and West of Scotland Branch *op.cit.*, minute book, 30 December 1912.
94. Hamilton (1981), 244.
95. *EMJ* [New Series] Vol. 10, February 1913, 98.
96. Little (1932) 330.
97. Printed annual report of the Forfarshire Medical Association *op.cit.*, 26 June 1913.
98. Glasgow Southern Medical Society *op.cit.*, minute book, 17 April 1913.
99. Glasgow Southern Medical Society *op.cit.*, minute book, 4 December 1913.

Conclusion

In the period after the Second World War and the introduction of the National Health Service, local medical societies continued, and today continue, to play an important role in the concerns of the Scottish medical profession. Despite, or because of, the enduring distinctions between various types of society; dining and social clubs, exclusive scientific and specialist associations, student medical and dental societies; a great number continue to thrive. Many of the remaining associations are 'general interest' societies which attract a wide membership with a mixture of eminent medical speakers, general medical discussion, and lively social events.

The role of women in medical societies has been slow to emerge in the more modern period, despite their gradual acceptance into the ranks of membership. Relatively few have become office bearers of societies. Louise McIlroy, elected Vice-President of the Glasgow Obstetrical and Gynacological Society in 1912,[1] and Winifred Wood, chosen as President of the Scottish Society of Anaesthetists in 1931, were early exceptions.[2] The appointment of Jean Herring, former chief obstetrician and gynaecologist at Maryfield Hospital, Dundee, as President of the Forfarshire Medical Association in 1966, was remarked on as a new departure.[3] Some societies and clubs, including the Scottish Midland and Western Medical Association, continue to bar female practitioners from membership.

Throughout the five chapters of this book there has been an oblique reference to the 'hidden agenda' of medical societies, in relation to discussions on pressing medical political problems of the day, but also in the field of local professional issues, for example, the 'fixing' of local University and hospital and public medical appointments, which went on outside the boundary of the written records of societies. The exclusive nature of some clubs and societies suggests that this may still occur, although it is more likely that present day deals are reached on the golf course rather than at representative meetings of the local profession in medical societies.

This book has sought to define the role of medical societies as a whole in the medical profession, rather than focus on the work of individual members or societies. In doing this, the educational, social, professional and political roles of Scottish medical societies have been discussed. Other areas, including the rise of speciality as reflected in the creation of new societies, and the changing relationship between local societies and the BMA, have also been considered. Yet this book serves only as an introduction to the subject: there is much that remains undone, a systematic comparison of Scottish societies with those in the rest of Britain in the period would undoubtedly provide new insight into the subject. It is also likely that some societies have remained undiscovered by this researcher, and that new evidence on the role of medical societies in professional development awaits analysis. This book is an exposition of the activities of 160 Scottish medical societies: future contributions are welcomed.

NOTES

1. At the time of her election Louise McIlroy was Assistant to the Muirhead Professor of Obstetrics and Gynaecology at Glasgow University and Assistant Surgeon in Gynaecology at Glasgow Royal Infirmary. *Medical Directory* 1913, 1348.
2. *Annals of the Scottish Society of Anaesthetists,* (1989), 19.
3. Blair (1990), 101.

Chronological List of Senior Scottish Medical Societies with Type Codes

NOTES

1. For more information on societies listed see individual alphabetical entries in part two of this book.
2. Societies marked with an asterisk were merged with another society or were re-formed at a later date.
3. Where there is some doubt over exact dates of formation or cessation first and last known dates of existence are prefixed < or suffixed >.
4. The abbreviation ext. is used to denote those societies which are still in existence. Unk. is used for societies where no probable date of demise has been established.
5. (E) denotes a society established in Edinburgh, (G) a society set up in Glasgow, and (I) identifies a society formed in Inverness.

Edinburgh Medical Society	1731–1737	1
Edinburgh Philosophical Society	1737–1783	3
Aberdeen Philosophical Society	1758–1773	3
Royal Physical Society (E)	1771–ext	3
Aesculapian Society (E)	1773–ext.	2
Dissipation Club (E)	<1782–unk.	2
Harveian Society (E)	1782–ext.	1
Royal Society of Edinburgh	1783–ext.	3
Gymnastic Society (E)	1786–1807	2
Aberdeen Medico-Chirurgical Society	1789–ext.	1
Glasgow Medical Club	1798–1814>	2
Chemical Society of Glasgow	1800–1801	3
Wernerian Natural History Society (E)	1808–1858	3
Glasgow Medical Society	1814–1866*	1
Royal Medico-Chirurgical Society of Glasgow*	*1814–ext.	1
Medical Society of the North (I)	1817–1829>	1
Greenock Medical and Chirurgical Association	1818–1851	1
Paisley Medical Society	1818–ext	1
Physico-Chemical Society of Edinburgh	1819–1822	3
Edinburgh Phrenological Society	1820–1870	3
Glasgow Medico-Chirurgical Society	1820–1832	1
Edinburgh Medico-Chirurgical Society	1821–ext.	1
Medico-Chirurgical Society of Dumfries	<1822–unk.	1
Lanark Medical Society	<1824–1827>	1
Dundee Phrenological Society	1825–1836>	3
Fife Medico-Chirurgical Society	1825–1840>	1
Glasgow Faculty of Medicine	1825–1904	1

Kilmarnock Phrenological Society	1826–1836>	3
Glasgow Phrenological Society	1829–1845	3
Anatomical Society of Edinburgh	1833–1845	1
Greenock Phrenological Society	1833–1836>	3
Cupar Phrenological Society	1835–1840>	3
Forfar Phrenological Society	1835–1836>	3
Aberdeen Phrenological Society	1836–1845>	3
Botanical Society of Edinburgh	1836–ext.	3
Statistical Society of Glasgow	1836–1843>	4
Stirling Medical Association	1836–1850>	1
Clackmannan and Kinross-shire Medical Association	1837–1917	1
Border Medical Society	1838–1878	1
Dumfries Phrenological Society	<1839–1840>	3
Eastern Medical Association of Scotland	1839–1841>	1
Western Medical Association	1839–1840>	1
Edinburgh Obstetrical Society	1840–ext.	5
Edinburgh Medical Missionary Society	1841–ext.	4
Granton Club (E)	1841–1853	2
Edinburgh and Glasgow Medical Club	1844–1851*	2
Glasgow Southern Medical Society	1844–ext.	1
Western Medical Club (G)	1845–ext.	2
Medical and Surgical Institute of Glasgow	1847–1851>	1
Edinburgh Royal Infirmary Clinical Society	<1849–unk.	1
Glasgow Pathological Society	1850–1854	5
Edinburgh Physiological Society	1851–1854>	5
Edinburgh Medico-Statistical Society	1852–1853>	5
Scottish Curative Mesmeric Association	1853–1862>	4
Garioch and Northern Medical Association	1854–1925	1
Central Medical Association	1856–1879	1
Edinburgh Medico-Chirurgical Club	<1858–unk.	2
Forfarshire Medical Association	1858–ext.	1
Association Scottish Medical Practitioners	1859–1861	7
Edinburgh Pathological Society	1859–1862	5
Glasgow Curative Mesmeric Association	1861–1862>	4
Menteith Medical Society	1861–unk.	1
Buchan Medical Society	1862–1935	1
Deeside Medical Association	<1863–1884>	1
Banff, Moray and Nairn Medical Association	1863–1872>	1
Northern Counties Medical Association	1863–1873	1
Dundee Medical Society	1864–1871*	1
Greenock Medical Society	1865–1903>	1
North of Scotland Medical Association	1865–1892	1
Inverness Medical Missionary Society	<1866–unk.	4
Aberdeen Medical Club	1868–1872	1
Glasgow and West of Scotland Medical Association	1868–1944*	4
Glasgow Medical Missionary Society	1868–1975>	4
Lothians Medical Association (E)	1868–1872	1
Royal Odonto-Chirurgical Society of Scotland	1868–ext.	5
Aberdeen Medical Missionary Society	<1869–1876>	4
Round Table Club (E)	1869–1895	2
Glasgow North Western Medical Society	1872–1876>	1
Scottish Midland and Western Medical Association	1872–ext.	1

Glasgow Pathological and Clinical Society	1873–1907*	1
Sanitary Association of Scotland*	1875–ext.	4
Caledonian Medical Society	1878*–1968	1
Perthshire Medical Association	1879–1888*	1
Society of Licentiates in Dental Surgery (G)	1880–unk.	5
Edinburgh Health Society	1881–1915	5
Glasgow Royal Infirmary Medical Society	1881–1894>	1
Dundee Medical Club	1882–ext.	2
Fifeshire Medical Association	1882–1932	1
Glasgow Obstetrical and Gynaecological Society	1885–ext.	5
Inverness Medical Society	1885–1906	1
Edinburgh Pathological Club	1886–ext.	1
Glasgow Microscopical Society	1886–1931*	3
Stirling Medical Society	1888–1909>	1
Edinburgh Royal Infirmary Residents' Club	1889–1908>	2
Scottish Microscopical Society	1889–1921	3
Belvedere Hospital Medical Society (G)	1890–1892>	1
Society Med. Officers of Health for Scotland	1891–1908*	7
Ayr and Prestwick Medical Society	<1892–1911>	1
Dundee Clinical Club	1893–1917	1
Glasgow Eastern Medical Society	1893–1933*	1
Town and Country Club (G)	1893–1896>	2
Scottish Medical Defence Association*	1895–1899	7
Western Infirmary Residents'·Club	1895–1935>	2
Scottish Poor Law Medical Officers' Association	1895–1946	7
Scottish Eastern Assoc. Medical Women*	1899–ext.	1
Galenian Society (E)	1900–unk.	1
Scottish Medico-Psychological Association	<1902–unk.	5
Glasgow Northern Medical Society	1902–1953	1
Glasgow Odontological Society	1902–1958>	5
Medical and Dental Defence Union of Scotland	1902–ext.	7
Glasgow, W of Scotland Assn Regd Medical Women*	1904–ext.	1
Glasgow Royal Infirmary Club	1907–1922>	2
Glasgow Western Medical Society*	1907–1925	1
Greenock Faculty of Medicine	1907–ext.	1
Edinburgh and Leith Medical Practitioners. Assn	1908–1931	1
Dundee Dental Club	1909–ext.	5
Scottish Otological and Laryngological Society	1910–1924>	6
Fifeshire Colliery Surgeons' Association	<1911–1916>	7
Govan Medical Society (G)	<1911–1927>	1
Association of School Medical Officers for Scotland	1911–1967*	7
Monklands Medical Society	<1913–1915>	1
Scottish Society of Anaesthetists	1914–ext.	6
Scottish Union of Medical Women	1919–1932	1
Scottish Opthalmological Club	1920–ext.	6
Scottish Branch, British Homoeopathic Society*	<1921–ext.	6
Glasgow Medical Lunch Club	1921–1922>	2
Scottish Association for Mental Health	1921–ext.	4
Scottish Thoracic Society	1921–ext.	5
Scottish Paediatric Society	1922–1972>	6
Edinburgh Clinical Club	1926–ext.	1
Glasgow Southern Women's Medical Society	<1927–1931>	1

Aberdeen and N of Scotland Assn of Medical Women	1927–1989	1
Journal Club (E)	1928–1939	2
Scottish Radiological Society	1936–ext.	6
Scottish Society for Experimental Medicine	1938–ext.	6

Chronological List of Scottish Student and Graduate Medical Societies

NOTE

(St A.) is the abbreviation for St Andrew's University. Other abbreviations are noted at the beginning of Appendix 1.

Royal Medical Society (E)	1737–ext.
Chirurgo–Medical Society (E)	1767–1782*
Physico–Chirurgical Society* (E)	1774–ext*
Medical Society of Aberdeen	<1768–1771>
Chirurgo–Obstetrical Society (E)	1786–1792>
Chirurgo–Physical Society (E)	1788–1796*
Aberdeen Medical Society*	1789–ext.
American Physical Society (E)	<1790–1796*
Hibernian Medical Society (E)	<1790–1799*
American Medical Society (E)	<1792–unk.
Hibernian Physical Society* (E)	<1792–unk.
Glasgow University Medico–Chirurgical Society	1802–ext.
Hunterian Medical Society (E)	1824–1868
Brown's Square Medical and Surgical Society (E)	1826–1827
Aberdeen University Medical Students' Society	1864–ext
St Mungo's College Medical Society (G)	1878–1914>
Dental Students' Association of Glasgow*	1880–ext.
Edinburgh Medical Students' Christian Association	<1887–unk.
Queen Margaret College Medical Society* (G)	1893–1969*
Glasgow University '88 Medical Club	1894–1907
Octogenarian Club (E)	1895–1939
Edinburgh University Physiological Society	1904–1913>
Edinburgh Women's Medical Society*	1913–1952
Bute Medical Society (St A.)	1915–ext.
St Andrew's University Medical Society	1916–unk.

Part Two

The Records of Scottish Medical Societies 1731–1939

Notes on the Lists of Scottish Medical Societies

1. < before or > after a date indicates that it is the first or last known reference to a society whose existence may pre- or post-date the reference.
2. A question mark after a date is included when there is some doubt as to the actual date of formation or demise of the society.
3. The following abbreviations have been used throughout the text:
   BMJ – *British Medical Journal*
   Ed.Al. – *Edinburgh Alamanac*. This is sometimes followed by e.g. (Western suppl.), which signifies the entry comes from the Western supplement section of the *Almanac*.
   EMJ – *Edinburgh Medical Journal*
   GMJ – *Glasgow Medical Journal*
   Med.Dir. – *Medical Directory*
   Year-Book – *The Year-Book of Scientific and Literary Societies of Great Britain and Ireland*.
4. Other abbreviations used in the text are:
   N.I. – None identified. This refers to publications and secondary sources.
   N.L. – None Located. Relates to society records.
   F.U. – Frequency Unknown. Relates to frequency of meetings.
5. The letter L in square brackets [L] is placed beside the title of those mixed membership societies which admitted interested lay persons as well as medical practitioners.
6. Where another medical society is referred to in a society entry this is followed by the entry number of the society in parenthesis. References to student societies in the main list have been identified as such. Senior society cross-references are identified separately in the student list.
7. An asterisk (*) is used to draw attention to some point of note in the title or date of existence of a society, which will be discussed in the text of the society's entry.
8. Frequency and times of meetings held refer to those in the period up to 1939 for societies which are still extant.
9. Where hospital and academic positions are listed for society members, these refer, where possible, to positions held at the time of the society's creation. More comprehensive career details are given for those persons who appear in more than one entry on the occasion of their first appearance and are cross-referenced thereafter.

Alphabetical List of Senior Scottish Medical Societies

1. Aberdeen and North of Scotland Association of Medical Women (1927–89)

History

The Association was set up as the northern Scottish representative body of the national Medical Women's Federation, which had been established in London in 1917. The Aberdeen and North of Scotland Association joined the Eastern and Western Associations, based in Edinburgh and Glasgow, who were original members of the Federation. Until 1932 when it was discontinued, the three Scottish associations acted together on local Scottish issues under the title of the Scottish Union of Medical Women (125). On its recent termination, members joined the Scottish Eastern branch of the MWF (111).

Objects

To hold clinical and social evenings. To defend the interests and employment opportunities of local female medical practitioners.

Membership

Open to all female practitioners in the area.

Meetings

Twice yearly, and as required.

Publications

N.I.

Records

N.L. See Wellcome Institute Library, London, Medical Women's Federation Archives, SA/MWF Council Minute book, 12 November 1927, 3 May 1929.

Secondary Sources

See quarterly *Newsletter of the Medical Women's Federation, passim.*

2. Aberdeen Medical Club (1868–75)

History

The Medical Club was set up as a social and educational club for a small clique of influential local practitioners. It gradually expanded its informal interests to include local medical political issues, e.g. appointments to Aberdeen Royal Infirmary. The Club was also instrumental in the creation of a local branch of the British Medical Association for Aberdeen, Banff and Kincardine district in 1872. Members included influential local medical practitioners, Alexander Ogston, later Regius Professor of Surgery at Aberdeen University and Surgeon at Aberdeen Royal Informary, and James W. F. Smith, Physician and Lecturer in Clinical Medicine at Aberdeen Royal Infirmary.

Objects

Club devised as a '... way of keeping up that harmony and friendship which should always exist among professional brethren'. (Medical Club minutes, 13 October 1868)

Membership

Always limited to four or five members.

Meetings

Monthly in a members' residence.

Publications

N.I.

Records

Minute Books 1868–75 in Manuscripts Collection, Aberdeen University Library.

Secondary Sources

N.I.

3. Aberdeen Medical Missionary Society (<1869–76) [L]

History

Aberdeen Medical Mission was one of several set up in the course of the 1860s, following the example of the Edinburgh Medical Missionary Society (37). Missionary societies differed from the majority of medical societies, in that they were charitable endeavours, formed to offer free medical treatment and dispensary facilities, and Christian instruction for those living in poor inner-city areas, and also for the purpose of training medical missionaries for work overseas. Those most involved in this medical service were medical students, although other medical practitioners were involved in the administration, and sometimes the provision of medical services to the poor.

Objects

To provide free medical service to the local poor and to train medical missionaries for service overseas.

Membership

Open to lay persons as well medical practitioners and medical students.

Meetings

Normally an annual business meeting to discuss the financial position of the mission and its dispensary facilities.

Publications

N.I.

Records

N.L.

Secondary Sources

Ed.Al. (Aberdeen suppl.) 1874, 41 and *passim.*
Glasgow Medical Examiner No. 9 (April 1870), 216.

4. Aberdeen Medico-Chirurgical Society (1789–extant)

History

The Society was set up by a group of 12 students under the original name of the Aberdeen Medical Society (see 1 in student list). The present title was assumed in 1811. At this date the society was divided into separate senior and junior sections open to qualified practitioners and students respectively. The Junior section was only intermittently active and was replaced by the Aberdeen University Medical Students' Society in 1864. The Senior section was much more significant and came to play an important role in the medical and public health concerns of the city. In 1818 for example, the managers of the Aberdeen Royal Infirmary contacted the society for advice on how to counteract the spread of 'contagious fever' in the city. The committee established to look into the epidemic produced a list of preventive measures which they recommended be included in a handbill and circulated locally at public expense. The Society completed the building of its own meeting hall in King Street in 1820, and it continued to meet there until 1973 when a new hall was opened at the Foresterhill medical complex. The society for many years possessed an extensive medical library (instituted in 1791), which held over 10,000 volumes when it was eventually sold in 1964. Only a small, primarily local, collection remains today.

Objects

To read papers on medical or medico-scientific subjects, and discuss local and national issues affecting the medical profession.

Membership

Open to all qualified, and later, all registered practitioners in Aberdeen and its environs. Relatively high membership costs compared to other societies, e.g. in 1860 the entrance fee was three guineas plus one guinea annual subscription. Average membership 1789–1939 was sixty-six, reaching a peak of 116 in 1935.

Meetings

On the first Thursday of each month at 8 p.m., during the Society's session running from November to July.

Publications

No transactions published. Occasionally printed fee tables for circulation in the local press and at chemist's shops.
Allardyce (1934).
Milne (1989).
Regulations of Aberdeen Medico-Chirurgical Society, With a List of Members. (Aberdeen, 1833).
Riddell (1922).

Records

Complete set of minute books, Aberdeen Medico-Chirurgical Library, Society Hall, Foresterhill, Aberdeen.

Secondary References

Craig, 'Aberdeen Medico-Chirurgical Society' (1937), 302–5.
Craig, 'Aberdeen Medico-Chirurgical Society' (1968) 5, 13.
Rodger (1893), *passim.*
Contemporary reports of Society meetings are to be found in *EMJ, BMJ* and *Lancet, passim.*
See also *Med.Dir.* and *Year-Book passim.*

5. Aberdeen Philosophical Society (1758–73*) [L]

History

A Society covering literary and scientific, as well as medical, interests. Also known as the 'Wise Club'. Members were University appointees (Marischal or King's Colleges) and/or members of the learned professions. Two of the six founder members were medical men, David Skene and John Gregory, Professor of Medicine at Kings College. (*The reformed nineteenth-century Philosophical Society did not give prominence to scientific medical debate, and is not included in the survey.)

Objects

To combine philosophical inquiry with conviviality.

Membership

Maximum number of members was limited to twelve at any one time and entry was subject to unanimous election. Membership fee was five shillings.

Meetings

In the rooms of local taverns on the second and fourth Tuesday of each month, at 2 p.m., preceded by lunch. One discourse to be delivered per month.

Publications

N.I. The revived Philosophical Society (1840–1939) published five volumes of Transactions.

Records

Minute books in Manuscripts Collection, Aberdeen University Library.

Secondary Sources

Aberdeen Philosophical Society Transactions Vol. 5 Pt. 7 (Aberdeen, 1938), *passim.*
Drummond 'Early Medical and Scientific Societies of North East Scotland' (1956–58), 31
Drummond, 'Early Medical and Scientific Societies' (1956), 243.
Ulman (Aberdeen, 1991).

6. Aberdeen Phrenological Society (1836–45>) [L]

History

The Aberdeen Phrenological Society was founded by James Straton, a local fishing tackle manufacturer. William Gregory, lecturer in Chemistry at King's College, Aberdeen, who later became Professor of Chemistry at Edinburgh University in 1844, and President of the Scottish Curative Mesmeric Association (124) in 1856, was a leading figure in the Society. Gregory was also a member of the Edinburgh Phrenological Society (46). Andrew Moir, extra-mural lecturer in anatomy in Aberdeen, was also a member of the APS. In 1838, he delivered lectures on anatomy and physiology before the Society.

Objects

To advance the interests of phrenological science. Straton's main preoccupation was with classifying heads, the 'mathematics of phrenology'.

Membership

Open to all interested in the science of phrenology, this and the other phrenological societies listed below represent those societies which included a significant medical presence in their ranks.

Meetings

F.U.

Publications

Articles by members of the Society appeared in the *Phrenological Journal, passim.*

Records

N.L.

Secondary Sources
Cooter (1984), 284, 287, 331n.
Cooter (1989), 1, 154, 203, 235, 317, 335.

7. Aesculapian Club (1773–extant)

History

The Aesculapian is a medical dining club, set up by Andrew Duncan Senior, an extramural lecturer in medicine in Edinburgh, and after 1789, Professor of the Institutes of Medicine at Edinburgh University (35, 40, 107). The Club was formed by Duncan in an attempt to encourage professional fellow-feeling through the promotion of convivial gatherings. A gold medal essay competition was instituted in 1777 for the best essay on a scientific subject submitted to the Club, but was discontinued the following year, and the social rather than the educational aspects of the club remained paramount. The recreational side of the Club extended to sporting contests, and frequent golf matches among the members led to the establishment of the off-shoot, Gymnastic Society (87), which was set up in 1786.

Objects

To cement the friendship between physicians and surgeons.

Membership

Open equally to physicians and surgeons. Membership limited to twenty-two.

Meetings

Originally, suppers were held on the first Friday of each month, later these were replaced by quarterly dinners held at various hotels.

Publications

Two private histories of the Club have been published:
Records of the 'Aesculapian' (1888, with suppl., 1906).
Stuart (1941).

Records

Minute books held in the Library of the Royal College of Physicians, Edinburgh.

Secondary Sources

EMJ 19/1 (1873), 563–72.
Guthrie 'Aesculapian Club of Edinburgh' (1967), 245–50.
Rolleston, 'Medical Friendships, Clubs and Societies' (1930), 254–5.

8. Anatomical Society of Edinburgh (1833–45)

History

Established in March 1833 by six medical practitioners in the city, including John Reid and James Young Simpson, Professor of Midwifery at Edinburgh University after 1840 (42, 93). John Goodsir, Professor of Anatomy at the University of Edinburgh, was President during its final year of existence. Members presented anatomical specimens accompanied by short verbal or written accounts of them. The Society was established at a time when the study of anatomy was expanding under the influence of Paris medical teaching in pathological anatomy, and many Edinburgh medical students, including Simpson, spent time in the Parisian medical schools. The Society's formulation also closely followed the creation of a chair of General Pathology at Edinburgh University in 1832, occupied by John Thomson.

Objects

'For the investigation of Animal and Vegetable Anatomy, Physiology, and Pathology'. (*Edinburgh Almanac*, 1835)

Membership

No indication as to the size of the Society. Candidates for admission had to possess a medical or surgical qualification.

Meetings

Fortnightly on the first and third Tuesday of each month at 8 p.m., at High School Yards, Surgeon's Square.

Publications

N.I.

Records

Minute book for 1833–43 in Manuscripts Collection, Edinburgh University Library.

Secondary Sources

Edinburgh Almanac (1835), 459, *passim.*
EMSJ 42 (1834), 367–79.
EMJ 19/2 (1874), 1018n.
Finlayson 'Records of Scientific and Medical Societies Preserved in the University Library, Edinburgh', *Bibliotheck* (1956–8), 15.
Maulitz (1987), 144–7 and *passim.*

9. Association of School Medical Officers for Scotland (1911–67*)

History

The Association was formed in the midst of several years of contentious debate (1909–12) over school board appointments in Scotland. Both the Glasgow Southern Medical Society (78) and the Glasgow and West of Scotland branch of the BMA took the step of expelling members (later reinstated) of their organisations who accepted such appointments which were viewed as a threat to general practitioners' private practice. The Association held its inaugural meeting in the offices of the Govan Parish School Board in Glasgow on 8 April 1911, attended by school medical officers from around the country. It was decided not to affiliate with any other existing society, but to remain an independent association. Medical matters of special relevance to SMO's were discussed, e.g. problems and treatment of ringworm. Included among the first council was a female practitioner, Kate Fraser, SMO for Govan Parish. The long-serving Honorary Secretary and Treasurer of the Society, (1916–39), was John Hunter, Medical Inspector of Schools for Linlithgow. The body became the Association of School Medical and Dental Officers in 1948. *In 1967, the Association was merged with the Scottish branch of the Society of Medical Officers of Health.

Objects

To protect the interests of SMO's and expand knowledge in the field of medical care in schools.

Membership

Open to medical practitioners holding school board appointments.

Meetings

Held around the country. Annual meeting in March.

Publications

N.I.

Records

N.L.

Secondary Sources

Lancet (1911), Pt. 1, 1234, 1301.
Med.Dir., passim.
Year-Book, (1921), 353 and *passim.*

10. Association of Scottish Medical Practitioners (1859–61)

History

Set up in Edinburgh in February 1859 to enforce the Clauses of the 1858 Medical Act, and in the wake of the Procurator Fiscal for Scotland's refusal to prosecute unregistered practitioners. The Association came to an abrupt end in January 1861 when it was discovered that the terms of the new Act did not make provision for recourse to law to protect the rights of qualified practitioners. The Association was the first attempt at organising the profession throughout Scotland.

Objects

To promote the enforcement of the Medical Act and to raise a fund to finance the prosecution of unregistered medical practitioners.

Membership

Open to all registered medical practitioners in Scotland. Membership fee was ten shillings.

Meetings

Inaugural meeting in Edinburgh attracted practitioners from as far and wide as Galashiels to Crieff, and Glasgow to St. Andrews. Local-sub committees were proposed for the larger Scottish towns.

Publications

N.I.

Records

N.L.

Secondary Sources

EMJ 5 (1859–60), 967; 6 (1860–61), 775

11. Ayr and Prestwick Medical Society* (<1892–1911>)

History

*The Society was initially known as the Ayrshire Medical Society and Club, but by 1907 had adopted the title of Ayr and Prestwick Medical Society. In 1911, its discussions of the implications of the National Health Insurance Bill were widely reported. The Society elected an Honorary President, who presented an annual address to the Society. In 1911, this was Sir David Caldwell McVail, then Crown Member for Scotland on the General Medical Council and Professor of Physiology and the Institutes of Medicine at Anderson's College Medical School.

Objects

To support the interests of the local profession, through regular meetings and social occasions.

Membership

Open to all practitioners in the area.

Meetings

Monthly in Ayr County Hospital. Held annual dinner.

Publications

N.I.

Records

N.L.

Secondary Sources
BMJ (1911), Pt. 2, 1439.
GMJ 77 (January–June 1912), 47.
Walker Downie (1923), 89.

12. Banff, Moray and Nairn Medical Association* (1863–72>)

History

The Association was one of the founder affiliate members of the North of Scotland Medical Association (100) in 1865, sending two delegates to the latter's annual conference in Aberdeen. Robert Turner of Keith, a council member of the BMNA in 1871 became President of the North of Scotland Association in 1873. *The Society was also sometimes referred to as the Elgin Medical Society, e.g. in the entries for the NSMA in the *Medical Directory*.

Objects

Fee-fixing and general concern for the status of the profession; no details of medical papers delivered.

Membership

No details of size or cost of membership; elected three office-bearers plus a six man council, from which two delegates were chosen to attend the annual meeting of the NSMA in Aberdeen.

Meetings

Half-yearly, in Elgin on last Saturday of January and July.

Publications

N.I.

Records

N.L. Printed table of fees dated January 30 1864 held among papers of Buchan Medical Society, Manuscripts Collection, Aberdeen University Library.

Secondary Sources

Med.Dir. (1868, 1871).

13. Belvedere Hospital Medical Society (1890–2)

History

One of many medical societies set up to meet the educational and social interests of medical staff in hospitals across Scotland. The Society at Belvedere Hospital, in the East End of Glasgow, apparently did not last long, since its books cover only a two year period. The social aspects of hospital association were however, revived between 1910 and 1914, in the form of a hospital golf club, whose records are retained alongside the Society's minute book (given below).

Objects

To provide a forum for educational exchange and social contact between the hospital's medical staff.

Membership

Open to medical staff of the hospital.

Publications

N.I.

Meetings

F.U.

Records

Society minute books in possession of Greater Glasgow Health Board Record Archive, University of Glasgow.

Secondary Sources

N.I.

14. Border Medical Society (1838–78)

History

This well-planned local society with a wide range of medical interests, was set up in Kelso in June 1838, with the intention of producing transactions of the Society's investigations into disease, local medical topography, and general medical papers. One volume of *Proceedings* exists published in Kelso in 1841, covering meetings held between 1839–41, but no other transactions have been located, although according to Hume (1853), up to three further volumes appeared.

Objects

The four main aims of the Society were: enquiry into the medical topography of the district; reading of papers on medical subjects; investigation into the causes and nature of disease in the district; and, the maintenance of the honour and respectability of the local profession.

Membership

Ordinary membership was open to qualified local practitioners, and in addition, provision was made for the admission of Corresponding and Honorary members. Annual subscription was five shillings. Membership numbers remained around twenty-four between 1838 and 1853, the last year for which figures are available.

Publications

Proceedings of the Border Medical Society (Kelso, 1841).

Meetings

Annually, initially in June, later changed to August, in different towns in the district by rotation.

Records

N.L.

Secondary Sources

EMJ 9 (1863–4), 677; 23/2 (1878), 1054.
Hume (1853), 192.
Med.Dir., passim.

15. *Botanical Society of Edinburgh (1836–extant)

History

Besides the hearing of papers, some later published in the Society's regular volumes of *Transactions*, the Society, in connection with the University of Edinburgh, instituted a herbarium, to which local and corresponding members contributed, and also possessed an extensive library. Regular field trips were, and are, an integral part of the Society's functions. For much of the nineteenth century the Society maintained a significant presence of medical practitioners, reinforcing the strong link between botany and medicine. Medical members today join through an interest in the subject. Meetings continue to be held in the Royal Botanical Gardens, with divisional meetings held around Scotland. *Reflecting the wider geographical spread of the its membership, the Society's title became the Botanical Society of Scotland in October 1991.

Objects

The promotion of botanical science and of other branches of natural history connected with it.

Membership

Members of the Society, known as 'Fellows', gained admission only after recommendation by two other Ordinary Fellows, and by securing the support of three-fourths of the electorate. Initial membership fees were half a guinea on admission and half a guinea annually. Non-resident Fellows made a single three-guinea payment. The Society, which in 1896 had a membership of 260 Fellows, also enjoyed the patronage of Queen Victoria.

Publications

Volumes of *Transactions of the Botanical Society of Edinburgh* have appeared at regular intervals since 1844. Occasional *Catalogues of Plants* and other single works were also printed.

Meetings

Monthly from November to July. Summer meetings at the Royal Botanical Gardens in Edinburgh, winter meetings in the Society's rooms in York Place.

Records

Minute books in Royal Botanical Gardens, Edinburgh.

Secondary Sources

Med.Dir,. passim.
Year-Book, passim.
Hume (1853), 182–3

16. Buchan Medical Society (1862–1935)

History

The Society was first convened on 5 August 1862 at Old Deer. At its second AGM the question of medical fees for the district was raised and tables of fees from other societies in the north of Scotland were examined. The following year, the Society laid down a schedule of fees to be followed by its members, which was published in the local press. Also in 1864, the Society first mooted the proposal for establishing a regional federation of northern medical societies, to meet on an annual basis in Aberdeen. The North of Scotland Medical Association (100) was set up the following year. The Society continued its strong medico-political interests, and at a special meeting called in June 1911, agreed to act according to the policy of the BMA in regard to the opposition of the medical profession to the proposed National Insurance legislation. No meetings of the Society were held between 1914 and 1919 due to the outbreak of the First World War, as was to be the case with many of the Scottish medical societies. After the war, the Society struggled vainly to increase its membership, and, after a seven-year gap 1928–34 when there were no meetings, the Buchan Medical Society held one final gathering in March 1935.

Objects

To read papers on medical subjects, to discuss medico-political issues of the day, to engender a fraternal professional atmosphere in the locality.

Membership

The average membership of the Society was eleven, reaching a peak of nineteen members in 1864. Membership fees were minimal, two shillings and sixpence in 1895, with an additional five shillings charged for the dinner traditionally held after the business part of the meeting.

Publications

N.I.

Meetings

Annually in August in various towns in the district. Additional special meetings were convened as required.

Records

The Society records are located in the Manuscripts Collection, Aberdeen University Library.

Secondary Sources

Med.Dir,. passim.
Gordon, 'Aberdeenshire Medical Associations' (1968), 3–5.
Year-Book (1884), 157 and *passim.*

17. Caledonian Medical Society (1878*–1968)

History

*The Caledonian Medical Society was first established as a student society by a small group of Highland medical students at the University of Edinburgh, which met briefly between February and April in 1878. The official date of formation is given in the Society's *Medical Directory* entries as 1881, when the Society was reconvened and its rules revised. The intention of the originators of the Society to promote the study of Celtic folk-medicine, ancient and contemporary, was continued as the Society expanded. For example, in 1902, a former President of the Society and joint Editor of the *Caledonian Medical Journal*, David Rorie, Parochial Medical Officer and Certified Factory Surgeon in Auchterderran in Fife (54), had two articles in the Journal, entitled 'The Scottish Bone Setter' and 'The Obstetric Folk-Lore of Fife'.

Objects

To share friendship and maintain comradeship between eligible medical graduates.

Membership

Open to University medical graduates of Highland descent. The Society had 20 members in 1885, and 36 in 1889. By 1906, the total membership was 232.

Publications

Caledonian Medical Journal printed quarterly 1883–1968.

Meetings

Annually, alternately in Scotland and England. Meeting included an address and dinner.

Records

Minute book of the Society for the years 1878–91 in the Library of the Royal College of Physicians, Glasgow.

Secondary Sources

BMJ (1901), Pt. 2, 489 and *passim.*
Caledonian Medical Journal, passim.
Milne (1989), 205.
Stirling Journal and Advertiser 20 July 1906, 4.
See also *Med.Dir.* and *Year-Book, passim.*

18. Central Medical Association of Scotland (1856–79)

History

In March 1860, the Association petitioned Parliament against the proposed amendment to the Registration of Deaths Act, Scotland, which the Association felt would have a detrimental effect on the income of the profession, with the onus placed on the profession, rather than relatives, to report deaths in their locality. The following year, John Mitchell Strachan, Parochial Medical Officer for Fossoway, former PMO for Dollar, and a Certified Factory Surgeon (20), was elected President of the Association, a position he held for the following decade. John Strachan was one of the leading figures behind the ambitious, but ultimately unsuccessful, proposal to establish a 'Scottish Medical Association' in the 1870s.

Objects

To promote the interests of the profession and good feeling among the members of the Association.

Membership

Open to all qualified practitioners residing in Central Scotland.

Publications

N.I.

Meetings

Annual general meeting in Stirling on the first Tuesday of September in a local hotel. Members dined together after the business meeting.

Records

N.L.

Secondary Sources

Ed.Al. (Western suppl.) (1861), 128 and *passim.*
Med.Dir,. passim.
Stirling Journal and Advertiser 18 September 1857, 2; 10 September 1858, 4; 10 October 1859, 4; 2 March 1860, 4.

19. Chemical Society of Glasgow (1800–1) [L]

History

The Society had its own rooms and laboratory in Graeme Street and was involved in practical chemistry, with experiments conducted weekly. The inaugural meeting was on 8 October 1800, but the first notice of a paper delivered before the Society did not occur until March 1801. This was an essay on the 'natural history, chemical attributes and medical uses of chemistry', by Robert Henderson. The inclusion of the medical applications of mercury in this paper highlights the link between medicine and chemical investigation at this time, although the list of members of the Society gives no indication of their occupations. No clue is given as to the reason for the Society's brief existence, although the cost of conducting experiments may have been a factor.

Objects

To conduct regular chemical experimentation, to furnish a laboratory suitable for this purpose, and to hear papers on chemical subjects.

Membership

Society began with twelve members, four others joined in the course of the year of its existence. The subscription fee was ten shillings, raised to one guinea in 1801, plus an additional one shilling per week to pay for the materials used to conduct experiments.

Publications
N.I.
Meetings
Weekly.
Records
Minutes/experiments book held in the University of Strathclyde Archives, Glasgow.
Secondary Sources
N.I.

20. Clackmannan and Kinross-shire Medical Association (1837–1917)

History

The Clackmannan Association was set up in Alloa in 1837. From the outset, the Society had a strong medico-political input, alongside its educational functions which included the purchase of the leading weekly and quarterly medical journals for circulation among the members. In 1840, the Society petitioned Parliament on the issue of medical reform, in the hopes of securing government recognition of legally qualified medical practitioners, and the outlawing of 'quacks'. Professional issues were tackled too, and in 1864, the Society devised a table of fees to be circulated in the area. In 1874, the Association was one of the prime movers, along with the Scottish Midland and Western Medical Association of Scotland (115), in the attempt to create a 'Scottish Medical Association'. John Mitchell Strachan, an office-bearer of both societies, (18) was elected a committee member of the Clackmannan Association's committee set up to promote the proposal, which ultimately failed.

Objects

To promote friendly discourse among the members; to advance medical science by the reading of papers; to circulate medical periodicals between members.

Membership

Open to all qualified practitioners living in the area.

Publications
N.I.
Meetings

Half-yearly, and as circumstances dictated, in various towns in the area. Later meetings were followed by dinner in a local hotel.

Records
N.L.
Secondary Sources
EMJ 20/1 (1874), 570.
Med.Dir,. passim.
Stirling Journal and Advertiser 15 May 1840, 4 and *passim.*
Year-Book (1884), 157 and *passim.*

21. Cupar Phrenological Society (1835–40>) [L]

History

The Society was instituted in August 1835. Two of the six medical practitioners in the town were members. By September 1836, the Society had amassed a sufficient number of heads and casts to furnish a museum. The Society also possessed a small library of phrenological and related works.

Objects

To further phrenological science by means of discussion and by the formation of a local phrenological museum.

Membership

Entrance fee five shillings. Membership stood at twenty in 1835.

Meetings

Fortnightly at Madras Academy, Cupar, for the reading of papers.

Publications

N.I.

Records

N.L. Part of the Society's collection of casts and death masks is retained in Cupar Museum.

Secondary References

Fife Herald 8 September 1836.
Leighton (1840), 23.
Cottrell Watson (1836), 121–2.

22. Deeside Medical Association (<1863–<84)

History

The Association was interested in the issue of medical remuneration, and in 1863, published its own tables of fees, to be circulated in the locality. The Society was also a member association of the North of Scotland Medical Association (100), sending its President and Secretary as delegates to the annual meeting in Aberdeen.

Objects

To promote local professional interests.

Membership

Open to all qualified medical practitioners practising on Deeside.

Meetings

F.U.

Publications

Printed table of fees, 1863, copy among the papers of the Buchan Medical Society, in the Manuscripts Collection, Aberdeen University Library.

Records

N.L.

Secondary References

Med.Dir., see entry for North of Scotland Medical Association, 1871, 806, and *passim.*

23. Dissipation Club (<1782–?)

History

This medical social club was in existence in the early 1780s and helped serve as a feeder organisation, along with the Aesculapian Club (7), to the Harveian Society of Edinburgh (35). The constitution of the Harveian noted that, '... those wishing to become members must be proposed at the April meeting of the Aesculapians or of the Dissipation Club in March'. Its title is suggestive of the animated social activity of the elite of the profession in eighteenth century Edinburgh, typified by the well-lubricated dinner in a local tavern.

Objects

To further professional fraternity through social activity.

Membership

Open to the medical professional elite of Edinburgh. Similar to that of the Harveian Society and the Aesculapian Club.

Meetings

F.U.

Publications

N.I.

Records

N.L.

Secondary References

Comrie, 'Edinburgh Harveian Society' (1937), 477.
Innes, 'Harveians of Edinburgh: Their First Two Hundred Years' (1983), 285.

24. Dumfries Phrenological Association (<1839–40>) [L]

History

Among the Society's membership were Ambrose and Archibald Blacklock. The former was Honorary Surgeon at Dumfries Infirmary, and curator of the DPS phrenological museum in 1840. Archibald Blacklock, a former Royal Naval Surgeon on the *Thames* in 1814, and Assistant Surgeon at the Royal Naval Hospital, Deal, was elected Vice-President of the Society in 1840. President of the Society in 1839 was Sir Andrew Halliday, who served as Consultant Physician at Crichton Royal Institute between 1838–39. A renowned lunacy reformer, he had published two works revealing the poor conditions of British lunatic institutions, and advocating the introduction of an asylum inspectorate. In 1841, William Alexander Francis Browne, Medical Superintendent of Crichton Royal Institute (1838–57), delivered a paper on the hereditary tendencies in mental disease before the DPS.

Objects

To further phrenological science. The establishment of a local phrenological museum.

Membership

Although it was open to all those interested in phrenology, the membership suggests a link between phrenological science and investigations into mental health among the medical members of the Society.

Meetings

F.U.

Publications

N.I.

Records

N.L.

Secondary References

Cooter (1989), 26, 106, 157.
Phrenological Journal 14 (1841), 221–31, 311–20, and *passim*.

25. Dundee Clinical Club (1893–1917)

History

Throughout the time of its existence, the Club met at the homes of each of its members in turn, with the host for the evening presiding over the meeting. It was the responsibility of the President of each meeting to ascertain what contributions were to be made at the meeting and to communicate the programme to the Secretary for circulation among other members of the Club seven days prior to the meeting. Medical guests were permitted to attend meetings of the Club, and frequently did so. Despite the limited membership of the Club, and notwithstanding the fact that meetings were held in member's homes, clinical patients were frequently shown to illustrate the case notes which were read. The Club's minutes are formalised and it is only on the occasion of the Club's 100th meeting in 1903, that comments on the generosity of the dinner and accompanying libations are recorded. The 200th meeting of the Club in April 1914 was afforded no such special reference, and thereafter the meetings of the Clinical Club became infrequent, and finally ceased altogether in December 1917 owing to the demands of war-time medical practice.

Objects

'… to facilitate the exchange of views on professional matters, to mutually help each other in the study and diagnosis of interesting cases, and for the reading and discussion of any papers a member was about to publish'. (Club Minutes, 21 July 1894)

Membership

Established with seven founder members, the Club remained a small group, with total membership figures amounting to sixteen. No set subscription fees were levied, the expenses of the Club at the end of each year were equally met by the members.

Meetings

Held monthly.

Publications

Rules of the Clinical Club (Dundee, 1899).

Records

Complete set of Minute books in the Archive Department, University of Dundee.

Secondary References

N.I.

26. Dundee Dental Club (1909–extant)

History

The inaugural meeting of the Club was held on 6 December 1909. The first President of the Dental Club was Walter Campbell, who had been an active member of the Dundee Medical Society (28), and his son, William Graham Campbell, became first Honorary Secretary. William Graham Campbell later became President of the Forfarshire Medical Association in 1923/4, delivering his Presidential Address on 'The Dundee Dental Hospital and Dental School'. At a meeting of the Club in November 1910, William Graham Campbell put forward the idea to establish a dental dispensary to serve the needs of the poor in the city. From this notion grew the scheme to fund a dental hospital in Dundee through the donations of local business men, which opened its doors in 1914. In 1916, St. Andrews University was granted permission to award the Licence in Dental Surgery, and in the same year a Dental School was set up in Dundee Dental Hospital, its lecturers appointed and recognised by the University. Although the initial intake of students was affected by the wartime situation, by 1919, the Dental School had forty five students. In 1920, an annual conjoint meeting of the Dundee Dental Club, the Glasgow

Odontological Society (73), and the Edinburgh-based Odonto-Chirurgical Society of Scotland (105), was inaugurated, and held in rotation in each of the three cities, with the local society acting as host on each occasion.

Objects

To create a professional focus for local dentists at a time when there was no institutional centre for dentists outside more general medical clubs and societies.

Membership

Open to all registered dental practitioners in the city.

Meetings

F.U.

Publications

N.I.

Records

Minute books held by the current Honorary Secretary, Dundee Dental Club.

Secondary References

Menzies Campbell (1958), 248.
W.G. Campbell, 'Dundee Dental Hospital and Dental School', *Transactions of the Forfarshire Medical Association* (Edinburgh, 1924), 5.

27. Dundee Medical Club (1882–extant)

History

The Dundee Medical Club was established in 1882, the year of the foundation of University College, Dundee, (although medical teaching was not established there until 1887). The Club had its origins in the occasional meetings of medical practitioners at the Dundee Medical Library which had been set up in 1880. Owing to the conviviality of such informal contact, the Medical Club was set up and from its outset the Club was chiefly concerned with the social side of professional interaction. In addition to meetings and an annual dinner, the Club held a picnic each year to which women were invited as guests, although no female medical practitioners were admitted into the Club until 1987. In 1901, the Club decided that admission should be restricted to practitioners who had resided in the district for five years, which suggests that the Club sought to maintain a degree of exclusivity at this time, although this was later reduced to one year, and non-practising medical appointees of University College, Dundee were exempted from this condition. Other social events have been organised by the Club, including lectures by guest medical speakers, and curling and theatre evenings, and an fishing tournament is held each year for members.

Objects

'for the lessening of that friction among members of our profession which so frequently occurs where individual interests are involved, and the provision of good fellowhip among the members of the medical profession in the neighbourhood'. (MS anonymous history of the Dundee Medical Club, among the Buist papers)

Membership

Open to qualified medical and dental practitioners in the area. Formed with eleven members, the annual subscription was two shillings and sixpence. In 1929 membership stood at eighty four.

Meetings

Initially on the first Saturday of each month at local hotels. By 1929, monthly meetings had given way to a Spring 'at Home' and a supper in the Autumn.

Publications

Rules of the Dundee Medical Club (Dundee, 1897).

Records

Minute books held by current Honorary Secretary, Dundee Medical Club. See also papers among the R. C. Buist Collection in Dundee Unversity Archives Department.

Secondary References

N.I.

28. Dundee Medical Society (*1864–71*)

History

The Society within two years of its formation had regular and relatively extensive reports of its medical and professional discussions reprinted in the *EMJ*. The Society met for a short time in its own rooms, but the failure to secure a permanent meeting place, may help account for the fact that it was short-lived. The last minuted entry was for December 1871, when the advisability of terminating the Society due to the small number of members attending its meetings was discussed. The failure of the Society perhaps also owed something to the prior existence of the thriving Forfarshire Medical Association (55) in the area.

The Society displayed a strong interest in professional and medico–political matters, as well as an awareness of contemporary medical scientific issues during its brief existence. In 1868, the case of a local practitioner who had acted as an unpaid medical witness at a court in Perth was discussed, while in March 1871, the President of the Society, William Lochart Gibson, Consultant Physican, Dundee Royal Infirmary, appealed to members to support the Adulteration of Food Amendment Bill which was to go before Parliament. In 1870, the various forms of anaesthesia were discussed and Walter Campbell, a dental surgeon, later President of the Dundee Dental Club (26), displayed the use of nitrous oxide gas in two dental extractions. *There had been a previous Dundee Medical Society, which existed briefly in 1829. Also, in 1894, there were attempts to revive the Society, but by this time the Dundee Medical Club (27) was also in existence. Both the Medical Club and the Forfarshire Medical Association continue to cater for the interests of the profession in the city.

Objects

To receive communications on medical and surgical topics; to hold meetings to converse on medical topics; to provide a library for the use of the members; and to promote professional improvement.

Membership

Open to all qualified medical practitioners in the city. Annual subscription fee was one guinea. The first formal meeting of the Society was attended by twelve members, and the combined membership of the Society during its seven year existence was thirty seven.

Meetings

On the first Wednesday of the month at 8.30 p.m., during the Society's session, which ran from November to April.

Publications

N.I.

Records

Minute book and other records held in the Archive Department, University of Dundee.

Secondary References
Blair (1990), 61.
EMJ 12 (1866–7), 756 and *passim*.
Med.Dir., *passim*.

29. Dundee Phrenological Society (1825–36>) [L]

History

The Dundee Phrenological Society was set up in August 1825. By 1836, it had healthy membership figures, a small museum, and a library containing 80 works on phrenological science.

Objects

The advance of phrenological science in the area.

Membership

Had reached a figure of between sixty and seventy members by 1835.

Meetings

F.U.

Publications

N.I.

Records

N.L.

Secondary References
Cooter (1984), 157; Cooter (1989), 106.
Watson (1836), 125.

30. Eastern Medical Association of Scotland (1839–41>)

History

The inaugural meeting of the Eastern Medical Association of Scotland was held on 8 December, 1839 in Dundee. Also known by the name of the East of Scotland Medical Association, this organisation was one of the first Scottish societies to demonstrate a strong interest in medical reform, and to consider the wider interests of the profession, outside the immediate local concerns of its membership. In 1840–1, the Eastern Society sent delegates to the London congresses on medical reform, held in Exeter Hall. These conferences, organised by the original British Medical Association, increased the parliamentary pressure for improved medical education, reform of the medical corporations, and the registration of qualified practitioners. The Association's joint-Secretaries, Alexander Webster (physician at Dundee Royal Infirmary), and John Livingstone, also became Corresponding members of the original BMA, whose President George Webster, was an Edinburgh graduate.

The Eastern Association corresponded with the Clackmannan and Kinross-shire Medical Association (20) in 1840, over the medical reform issue, and the CKMA sent a delegates to the Association's meeting in Perth in January 1841. The Association also set up a committee, convened by Alexander Keiller (Physician at Edinburgh Royal Infirmary, and extra-mural Lecturer in Medical Jurisprudence at Edinburgh University) to consider the question of fixing a standard fee code for its members, but the proposal failed due to the great disparity in fees charged among its membership.

Objects

Formed for the purpose of medical reform and promoting professional medical interests.

Membership

Open to qualified practitioners residing in the counties of Forfar, Perth, and Fife.

Meetings

F.U.

Publications

N.I.

Records

N.L.

Secondary References

EMJ 12 (1866–7), 958.
Little (1932), 35–6.
McMenemy (1959), 197, 212–13, 218.
Provincial Medical and Surgical Association Journal (later *BMJ*), January 1841, 236–8.
Stirling Journal and Advertiser 15 May, 1840, 4; 26 June 1840, 4.
Waddington (1984), 72–3.

31. Edinburgh and Glasgow Medical Club (1844–51, 1890–1911>*)

History

A social club open to practitioners from Scotland's two largest cities and their environs. Meetings took the form of an afternoon excursion to a place of interest in or near the host city, followed by a dinner. *Although the original Club ended in 1851, it was revived in November 1890, by Sir Andrew Douglas Maclagan (Professor of Medical Jurisprudence at Edinburgh University), one of the founder members of the original society (he graduated MD at Edinburgh in 1833) and William Tennant Gairdner (see also 39, 41, 47, 50, 74), Physician in Ordinary to the Queen in Scotland, and Professor of Medicine at Glasgow University. Gairdner was a former Pathologist and Assistant Physician at the Edinburgh Royal Infirmary, one of many medical practitioners who moved from one city to the other in the course of their careers. The reformed Club held its 20th annual dinner in 1911.

Objects

To augment friendly relations between medical men in Glasgow and Edinburgh.

Membership

Open to equal numbers of practitioners from the East and West of Scotland. Original members were drawn chiefly from the elite of the profession, i.e. those holding university or hospital appointments.

Meetings

Twice yearly, in winter and summer. Held alternately in Edinburgh and Glasgow. The reconstituted Club met annually.

Publications

N.I.

Records

Minute book for 1844–51 held in the Library of the Royal College of Physicians, Edinburgh.

Secondary References

BMJ (1901) Pt. 2, 489; (1911), Pt. 1, 395.
Dow and Calman (1991), 72.
Gibson (1912), 276–7.

32. Edinburgh and Leith Medical Practitioners Association (1908–31)

History

This Society, first launched in 1908 to act in matters affecting local practitioners, was given new impetus during the profession's struggle against the National Insurance Act. Referred to in 1912 as the Leith Medical Practitioners' Association (Leith was not within the city boundary at this time), there is a suggestion that, despite comments to the contrary in the *BMJ* and *EMJ*, there was some degree of friction between local Leith practitioners, and the actions of the larger Edinburgh-based medical societies, including possibly the BMA branch. This is supported by the fact that by 1912, all medical practitioners in Leith had joined the Society. Any such unidentified dispute may have been short-lived, since subsequent references give the Association its full title.

Objects

'To promote and safeguard the interests of the medical profession.' (Quoted in notice of the Society's intentions in *BMJ* 16 March 1912)

Membership

Open to practitioners in the city of Edinburgh, and the burgh of Leith.

Meetings

Irregular. Originally held in the Hall of the Royal Medical Society (student society entry 23) Annual meeting in October.

Publications

N.I.

Records

N.L.

Secondary References

BMJ (1910), Pt. 1, 286; (1912), Pt. 1, 641.
EMJ [New series] 2 (1908), 293; 8 (1912), 291.
Lancet (1908), Pt. 2, 1185.
Year-Book (1913), 370 and *passim*.

33. Edinburgh Clinical Club (1926–extant)

History

This Club was set up in February 1926 in direct response to the needs of general practitioners in the city, some of whom felt that existing societies in the city were not catering for the interests and preoccupations of local general practitioners. The Club provides medical discussions, demonstrations, and hospital visits, in a more relaxed atmosphere than the formal settings of the older medical societies in Edinburgh.

Objects

To discuss a wide range of medical matters of interest to, or affecting, general practitioners.

Membership

The Club began with around fifty members, reaching a peak of over 100 in 1946. There are currently thirty members. Initial subscriptions were five shillings, and are presently £7 per year.

Meetings

On the third Tuesday of every month.

Publications

N.I.

Records

Minute books held by the Edinburgh Clinical Club.

Secondary References

N.I.

34. Edinburgh Galenian Society (1900–?)

History

The Society was established by ten junior members of the Edinburgh Medico-Chirurgical Society (40) in 1900. Members were University of Edinburgh junior medical assistants, and Clinical tutors. The discussions were reputedly of a high standard, and subsequently, six of the members of the Society were appointed to University chairs.

Objects

To provide greater opportunities for medical discussion for younger practitioners than was available in the Edinburgh Medico-Chirurgical Society.

Membership

Membership was originally ten, but was later expanded to sixteen.

Meetings

F.U.

Publications

N.I.

Records

N.L. See Edinburgh Medico-Chirurgical Society records, letter from Professor Edwin Bramwell, former Professor of Clinical Medicine at Edinburgh University, to the Society, 6 November 1946 (MAC GD 3/5/9/3/1).

Secondary References

N.I.

35. Edinburgh Harveian Society (1782–extant)

History

The idea for the Harveian Society, or Circulation Club as it was also known until 1829, came from Andrew Duncan Senior, who was also behind the setting up of the Aesculapian Club (7), in 1773, and the Edinburgh Medico-Chirurgical Society in 1821 (40). Duncan envisioned a larger club than the numerically limited Aesculapian, to take over the expense of running the prize essay competition for medical students which had been instituted in 1777, and to establish an annual festival to commemorate renowned medical figures. Duncan remained Secretary of the Society for forty six years until his death in 1828. Early features of the Society dinners were wagers between members to ensure a continued supply of drinks for all, and entertainment in the form of songs and poems. The prize essay competition continued at irregular intervals until 1865 when it was discontinued. After the Second World War membership of the Society was opened to include medical practitioners from across Scotland.

Objects

To hold an annual oration and dinner celebrating the 'discovery of circulation by the circulation of the glass'.

Membership

Initially set at 30 members, later became unlimited, and was finally fixed at 240 in 1963. Open to members of the college of physicians or surgeons in Edinburgh, and later to medical graduates of the University of Edinburgh. Original subscription fee was 6 shillings.

Meetings

For many years the annual dinner with oration was held annually on the anniversary of the birth of William Harvey, 12 April. It is now held in June of each year. The 'Harveian Festival' was originally celebrated at various taverns and hotels in the city, but found a permanent home in the hall of the Royal College of Physicians, Edinburgh.

Publications

Various Harveian orations were published, and copies are held in Edinburgh University Library. The first was 'An account of... the late John Hope... delivered as the Harveian Oration at Edinburgh for the Year 1788' by Andrew Duncan Senior, (Edinburgh, 1788).

Records

Minute books in the Royal College of Physicians, Edinburgh.

Secondary References

BMJ (1895) pt. 1, 28–9, and *passim.*
Comrie, 'Edinburgh Harveian Society' (1937), 476–9.
EMSJ 5 (1809), 386, and *passim.*
EMJ 20/1 (1874), 97–104; 8 (New series) (1912), 101–22 and *passim.*
Guthrie, 'Harveian Tradition in Scotland' (1957), 120–5.
Innes, 'Harveians of Edinburgh – Their first two hundred years' (1983), 285–9.
Medical Press and Circular 195 (1937), 476–9.
Power, *British Medical Societies* (1939), 45–52.
Watson-Wemyss (1933).
Year-Book, passim.

36. Edinburgh Health Society (1881–1915) [L]

History

The Edinburgh Health Society was formed at a time when the poor general health of the population was causing national concern. Under the Presidency of former Liberal Prime Minister, Lord Rosebery, between 1899 and 1915, the Society aimed to improve the health of the nation by increased awareness of the threat of disease and information on preventive measures which could be taken.

Objects

'To inculcate the laws of health' to the wider population.

Membership

Open to those interested in matters of health. The vast majority of the lectures were delivered by medical practitioners. Membership cost was 1 shilling per week. Life membership was one pound one shilling.

Meetings

Weekly during the months of November and December until 1901, when regular meetings ceased, although the Society continued its existence until 1915.

Publications

Published a series of penny and two penny pamphlets based on the lectures delivered before the Society; e.g. 'The Prevention of Consumption: Personal and Citizen Responsibility', by R.W. Philip (1900).

Records

N.I.

Secondary References
Ed.Al. (1900), 1114, *passim.*
Year-Book (1900), 269, *passim.*

37. Edinburgh Medical Missionary Society (1841–extant) [L]

History

The Society began as 'Edinburgh Association for sending Medical Aid to foreign countries' in November 1841. The Committee comprised leading medical and church figures, including: Thomas Chalmers, the Professor of Theology at Edinburgh University; William Pulteney Alison, Professor of the Practice of Physic; and James Syme, Professor of Surgery. In 1842, overtures were made to medical students to consider taking up medical missionary work, and a series of six weekly lectures was inaugurated at the University medical school. Medical missionary work was extended to the poorer communities of Edinburgh in 1853, under the auspices of Dr. Peter Handyside, lecturer in the College of Surgery. This home medical mission aspect of the Society's philanthropic activity grew, and a succession of medical students gained practical work experience in the mission dispensary in the Cowgate area of the city, which remained open until the introduction of the National Health Service reforms in 1948.

Objects

To train medical students for missionary work overseas and at home.

Membership

Open to medical practitioners, students, and interested members of the Church of Scotland.

Meetings

F.U.

Publications

Annual Reports; Occasional Papers (1854–9); *Quarterly Papers* (1871–1941>), *etc.*

Records

In the Overseas Medical Mission House, Edinburgh.

Secondary References
Checkland (1980), 80–2.
EMJ 3 (1857–8), 572–4, and *passim.*
Lechmere-Taylor (1941).
Lowe (1886), *passim.*
See also *Med.Dir* and *Year-Book, passim.*

38. Edinburgh Medical Society (1731–7*)

History

The Society was founded by the medical professors at the University of Edinburgh, plus nine other Edinburgh physicians and surgeons. It did not remain as an active group for long, ceasing to meet soon after the publication of the first volume of *Essays* in 1732. The Society was dominated by its Secretary, Alexander Monro *primus*, Professor of Anatomy. He undertook the editing of the *Essays*, which featured many articles by Monro, and by his son, Alexander Monro *secundus*, who succeeded him as Professor of Anatomy at the University of Edinburgh. The Society was superseded in 1737, by the Edinburgh Philosophical Society (45), which continued to publish medical contributions in its *Transactions*.

Objects

To discuss and publish cases received in the Royal Infirmary of Edinburgh. This was soon expanded to hear essays on all medical topics.

Membership

Active membership was confined to Edinburgh medical practitioners, but contributions from around Scotland, and from England, Ireland and the Colonies, were included in the published *Essays*.

Meetings

Monthly meetings were held at which papers were read between 1732–3. After this time papers were communicated to the Society for editing by Monro *primus*.

Publications

Five volumes of *Medical Essays* were published in Edinburgh between 1732–7, these went through five British editions and were translated into French, Dutch and German.

Records

N.L.

Secondary References

Emerson, 'Philosophical Society of Edinburgh 1737–1747' (1979), 151–91. (The first of a series of articles on the Philosophical Society, (45).)
EMSJ 75 (1851), 447–51.
Erlam, 'Alexander Monro, *primus*' (1953–5), 77–105.
McElroy (1969), 30.
Wright-St.Clair (1974), *passim*.

39. Edinburgh Medico-Chirurgical Club (<1858–?)

History

One in a long line of elite medical dining clubs established in Edinburgh. William Tennant Gairdner, (31, 41, 47, 50, 74), was elected a member in 1858, at the early age of 34. The Club was presumably an off-shoot of the senior Society of the same title (40).

Objects

To hold regular dinners and further professional understanding.

Membership

Limited to twenty. Club membership conferred on leading Edinburgh physicians and surgeons.

Meetings

Dinners three times annually.

Publications

N.I.

Records

N.L.

Secondary References

Gibson (1912), 273.

40. Edinburgh Medico-Chirurgical Society (1821–extant)

History

The Edinburgh Medico-Chirurgical Society was set up in May 1821, with fifty three original members. Its constitution and aims were based on those of the Medico-

Chirurgical Society of London. Andrew Duncan Senior (7, 35, 107) was the Society's first President, and Robert Hamilton (46), the first Secretary. From its outset, the Society had strong interests in furthering medical science. In 1831, a plan was drawn up to collect and collate medical cases from among its members and other willing practitioners, to be compiled into volumes dealing with specific branches of medicine and surgery, which would then be published and made available to the profession generally. In 1834, the first fruits of this project were published in the *Edinburgh Medical and Surgical Journal*, dealing with 'Diseases of the Brain and Nerves'. Although this series of case histories was not followed up, complete reports of the Society's proceedings were published on a regular basis in the *EMSJ* (soon to become the *EMJ*), from 1855.

Objects

'To receive and discuss communications on medicine, surgery and the allied sciences... and to promote professional improvement by any other means that may, from time to time, be approved of by the Society.' (Reprinted Laws of the Society, 1869)

Membership

Open to all qualified medical practitioners in the city. A category of corresponding membership, open to practitioners from elsewhere in Scotland, and from Europe and the Colonies, was also established in 1821.

Meetings

Monthly, on the first Wednesday of the month, at 8 p.m. from November to July.

Publications

Transactions published at irregular intervals. First volume appeared in 1824.

Records

In Special Collections, Edinburgh University Library.

Secondary References

EMSJ 17 (1821), 637; 42 (1834), 237–92; 82 (1855), 141–6 and *passim*.
EMJ 19/2 (1874), 769–87; 895–912; 1004–20; 1092–1105, and *passim*.
Edinburgh Almanac, passim.
Monthly Journal of Medical Science 10 (1850), 78–80.
See also *Med.Dir.* and *Year-Book, passim*.

41. Edinburgh Medico-Statitistical Association (1852–3?)

History

The Association grew out of a scheme for the registration of deaths in Edinburgh initially undertaken by the Edinburgh Medico-Chirurgical Society (40). William Tennant Gairdner (31, 39, 47, 50, 74) and John Warburton Begbie (Physician at New Town Dispensary), were joint Secretaries and Registrars. The first and probably, only report of the Association considered seventy five patient deaths, details of which had been supplied by twenty three practitioners in Edinburgh and Leith. The patient deaths were recorded in terms of sex, marital condition, place of residence, age, place of death, position in society (in status categories devised by the Association), and there was a separate detailed section on causes of death. There is no clear evidence as to the fate of the Association, no further meetings are recorded in the *Monthly Journal of Medical Science* after the inclusion of the twelve page Annual Report for 1852, and it is possible that medical statistical enquiry in Edinburgh was continued under the auspices of the Edinburgh Medico-Chirirurgical Society.

Objects

To provide statistical background to the patterns of disease and mortality in the city of Edinburgh.

Membership

Open to all practitioners residing in Edinburgh with an interest in medical statistics. Twenty-three members in 1852.

Meetings

Quarterly.

Publications

First Report of the Medico–Statistical Association (Edinburgh, 1852).

Records

N.L.

Secondary References

Gibson (1912), 55.
Monthly Journal of Medical Science 14 (January–June 1852), 580; 15 (July–December 1852), 288–99.

42. Edinburgh Obstetrical Society (1840–extant)

History

The Society was established by local practitioners with the intention of increasing the status of obstetrics within medical practice. Although an increasingly integral part of general practice, midwifery and obstetrical service was not regarded as a significant aspect of medical instruction or science in the first decades of the nineteenth century. The Edinburgh Obstetrical Society, and its earlier counterparts in London, and Dublin, helped improve the position of obstetrical and gynaecological practice and investigation. James Young Simpson (8, 93) was for many years the leading figure in the Society, as President (1841–58) and leading contributor to both the Society's discussions and its early volumes of proceedings. The Society granted qualified female practitioners membership in 1893, and was one of the first Scottish medical societies to do so.

Objects

'... to advance Obstetrical Medicine, by holding meetings for the purpose of receiving communications and conversing on subjects connected with that branch of the profession.' (Laws of the Society, 1840)

Membership

Open to those engaged in the practice of midwifery, and in possession of a medical or surgical qualification. Formed with twenty members, figures soon increased, and in the period down to 1939 reached an average of 159, peaking at 245 in 1895. (This figure does not include the non-resident Fellows of the Society who were listed as Ordinary Fellows alongside local members in the Society's *Transactions* after 1870). The original entrance fee was one guinea, with a further five shillings annual contribution.

Meetings

On the third Wednesday of each month at 8 p.m.

Publications

Transactions published irregularly. A single volume of proceedings based on journal reports was published in 1848, and the first volume of *Transactions of the Obstetrical Society of Edinburgh* appeared in 1870. After 1880 annual *Transactions* appeared.

Records

Incomplete run of minute books in the Royal College of Physicians, Edinburgh.

Secondary References

BMJ (1895), Pt. 2, 133 and *passim*.

See *EMJ* 35/2 (1890), 738–47, 831–44, and *passim.*
Med.Dir. 1853, 784–5 *and passim.*
Monthly Journal of Medical Science, 1848 and *passim,*
Year-Book, passim,

43. Edinburgh Pathological Club (1886–extant*)

History

Set up by Sir John Batty Tuke (then Visiting Physician at Saughton Hall Private Asylum, and Lecturer on Insanity and Mental Disease at the Royal College of Physicians and the the Royal College of Surgeons in Edinburgh), at a dinner party for medical associates held at his house. The Club was purposely not established as a formal society, and there are no office bearers other than the Secretary. At meetings, the Chair is taken by the third person entering the room, and no paper is allowed to exceed thirty minutes duration. The Club's first Secretary was German Sims Woodhead, then Pathologist at Edinburgh Royal Infirmary and Demonstrator in Pathology at Edinburgh University. Sims Woodhead founded the *Journal of Pathology and Bacteriology* and was elected professor of Pathology at Cambridge University in 1890. The Club heard subjects on a wide range of medical subjects, including several on veterinary medicine, (among the ranks of the Club were members of the Faculty of Veterinary Medicine). The Club was active in the field of medical education and a series of special meetings in 1908 led to the private publication of two reports on the subject in 1909. Unlike many other Scottish medical societies, the Club continued to meeting throughout the period of the First World War, and these meetings included a further series on the position of medical education at Edinburgh University. *The Club no longer meets on a regular basis.

Objects

Originally set up to discuss, through short papers, subjects connected with pathology; in practice general medical matters were also discussed.

Membership

At first limited to twenty-five members, this was soon expanded, and in 1900, thirty three members attended the 100th meeting of the Club. The Club reached a membership of ninety-two in 1954, and in 1968 it stood at 265. Annual subscription was originally five shillings.

Meetings

Monthly.

Publications

An Inquiry into the Medical Curriculum (Edinburgh, 1909).

Records

Held by the current Secretary of the Edinburgh Pathological Club.

Secondary References

See *EMJ, passim.*
Guthrie, 'The Edinburgh Pathological Club' (1966), 87–91.

44. Edinburgh Pathological Society (1859–62)

History

This Society had strong links with the University of Edinburgh, and included among its Honorary Members all the then Professors of the Medical Faculty. No information on reasons for its demise has been obtained.

Objects

The cultivation of pathology and morbid anatomy.

Membership

Open to all medical practitioners, and Professors and students of the Faculty of Medicine, University of Edinburgh. Members were elected by ballot at the Annual General Meeting.

Meetings

Monthly from November to July.

Publications

N.I.

Records

N.L.

Secondary References

Med.Dir. (1861), 826, and (1862), 800.

45. Edinburgh Philosophical Society (1737–83*) [L]

History

The Philosophical Society (full title: Society for Improving Arts and Sciences, and particularly Natural Knowledge) had its origins in the demise of the Edinburgh Medical Society (38) in 1737. Although the remit of the new Society was broader, covering science and philosophy, medical representation remained strong both in terms of membership figures, and particularly, in contributions to the Society's transactions. Many of the Philosophical Society's original medical members had been involved with the earlier society. A limit of one third of over-all membership was allocated for members outside the fields of medicine and philosophty. The great majority of papers included in all three volumes of Society transactions were on medical subjects. *The Society was reconstituted as the Royal Society of Edinburgh (107) in 1783.

Objects

The improvement of arts and sciences through enquiry and experimentation.

Membership

Sixteen of the forty eight members in 1739 were medical practitioners. Annual membership fee was one giunea.

Meetings

On the first Thursday of every month, at 4 p.m.

Publications

Essays and Observations, Physical and Literary 3 vols, (Edinburgh, 1754, 1756, 1771).

Records

N.L.

Secondary References

Emerson, 'Philosophical Society of Edinburgh 1737–1747' (1979), 151–91.

——, 'Philosophical Society of Edinburgh 1748–1768' (1981), 133–76.

——, 'Philosophical Society of Edinburgh 1768–1783' (1985), 255–303.

——, 'The Scottish Enlightenment and the end of the Philosophical Society of Edinburgh' (1988), 33–66.

——, 'Science and the Origins and Concerns of the Scottish Enlightenment' (1988), 333–66.

——, 'Sir Robert Sibbald, Kt, the Royal Society of Scotland and the Origins of the Scottish Enlightenment' (1988), 41–72.

46. Edinburgh Phrenological Soceity (1820–70) [L]

History

Closely modelled on other scientific and medico-scientific societies of the time, the Phrenological Society initially met in the University of Edinburgh. No members of the Medical Faculty joined the Society, although medical students and practitioners in the city became members (seven qualified medical practitioners were members in 1840). Robert Hamilton, one of the founders of the Edinburgh Medico-Chirurgical Society (40) was Vice-President of the Society in 1821. The creation of a phrenological museum was one of the Society's main intentions, and this collection was displayed in the Society's purpose-built museum in Chambers Street until the Society's demise. Parts of the collection remain today in the museum of the University's Anatomy Department. By 1840, the Society had become less interested in promoting the science of phrenology through the presentation of papers, than in its wider natural history aspects, chiefly through its collection of casts and skulls.

Objects

'... to hear papers, and to discuss questions connected with phrenology; to hold a correspondence with Societies who take an interest in the System; and thus, to collect and preserve, facts and views, that may improve and enlarge the boundaries of science.' (Laws of the Phrenological Society, 1820)

Membership

Admission fee was two guineas, plus one guinea annually. Society established by six founding members, membership stood at fifty one in 1840.

Meetings

Fortnightly on Tuesdays at 8 p.m. between November and April.

Publications

Transactions of the Edinburgh Phrenological Society (Edinburgh, 1823).
Phrenological Journal 10 vols (1824–47).

Records

Minute and letter-books held in Special Collections, Edinburgh University Library.

Secondary References

Combe (1850), *passim.*
Cooter (1984), 79 and *passim.*
Cooter (1989), 114–16 and *passim.*
EMJ 19/2 (1874), 770.
Finlayson, 'Records of Scientific and Medical Societies preserved in the University Library Edinburgh: Additions' (1963–6), 38.
Phrenological Journal, passim.
Cottrell Watson (1836), *passim.*
See *Med.Dir.* and *Ed.Al,. passim.*

47. Edinburgh Physiological Society (1851–4>)

History

Reports of the Physiological Society's meetings were included in the *Monthly Journal Of Medical Science* between 1851 and its end in 1853, at which time the Journal was merged with the *EMSJ*, and appeared in 1855 as the *EMJ*. President of the Society throughout this period was John Hughes Bennett, Professor of the Theory of Physic and Clinical Medicine at the University of Edinburgh (93). Meetings of the Society consisted in the display of dissections and drawings of human and animal specimens, and the delivery of papers and case notes. William Tennant Gairdner, then Pathologist at Edinburgh Royal Infirmary, (31, 39, 41, 50, 74) was Vice-President of the Society in the years 1853–4.

Objects

The investigation of the structure and functions of beings.

Membership

Open to all interested qualified practitioners and students.

Meetings

Fortnightly in Edinburgh University.

Publications

N.I.

Records

N.L.

Secondary References

Med.Dir. 1854.
Monthly Journal of Medical Science 14 (January–June 1852), 281–7, and *passim*.

48. Edinburgh Round Table Club (1869–95)

History

One in a long line of Edinburgh medical social clubs. The Club met regularly in Edinburgh hotels for dinner, and also made summer excursions to local places of interest for picnics and to play bowls and golf. Among the founding members were Professors Alexander Dixon, John Chiene, Thomas Annandale, Arthur Gamgee, and William Rutherford.

Objects

To promote good fellowship among its members.

Membership

Limited to a maximum of twenty at any given time. Established with ten members, had sixteen members in 1870.

Meetings

Three per year.

Publications

N.I.

Records

Minute books and other records in Special Collections, Edinburgh University Library.

Secondary References

Bayliss, 'Round Table Club, Edinburgh' (1980), 438–40.
Chiene, *Looking Back: 1907–1860* (1907), 38.
Finlayson (1956–8), 18.
Miller, 'Let the Bow be Unstrung' 105 (1976), 272–6.
McKendrick (1908).
Rolleston, 'Medical Friendships, Clubs and Societies' (1930), 255.

49. Edinburgh Royal Infirmary Clinical Society (<1849–?)

History

Little is known of this Society other than the title of two papers presented before it by a former ship's surgeon, Thomas Stratton on '[health on] emigrant ships to North America' and the 'History of epidemic cholera in Chatam, Rochester and Stroud'. These papers were subsequently printed in the *Edinburgh Medical and Surgical Journal* in 1850 and 1851.

Objects

To hear papers on clinical subjects.

Membership

Open to clinical staff of Edinburgh Royal Infirmary.

Meetings

F.U.

Publications

N.I.

Records

N.L.

Secondary References

EMSJ 73 (1850), 33 and *passim*; 75 (1851), 253 and *passim*.

50. Edinburgh Royal Infirmary Residents' Club (1889–1908>)

History

A social club for resident physicians and surgeons of Edinburgh Royal Infirmary. The Club held annual dinners, attended by past and present residents, some of whom had risen to eminence in the profession, including William Tennant Gairdner (31, 39, 41, 47, 74). Other prominent medical figures also attended the Club's official functions e.g. in 1907, John Yellowlees, Honorary Consultant Physician at Glasgow Royal Asylum at Gartnavel and former Resident Physician at Edinburgh Royal Infirmary, attended the annual dinner.

Objects

To promote and maintain friendship among the current and former resident medical staff of the Infirmary.

Membership

Open to past and present residents of Edinburgh Royal Infirmary.

Meetings

F.U. Annual dinner.

Publications

N.I.

Records

N.L.

Secondary References

EMJ 2 [New series] (1908), 101.
Gray (1952), 252.
Gibson (1912), 158.

51. Edinburgh Royal Physical Society (1771–extant) [L]

History

Originally a small student society (entry 21 in student and graduate list), the Physical Society soon benefited from its union with several other student medical societies in the course of the late eighteenth and early nineteenth centuries. For the first fifty years of its existence the President of the Society was a medical graduate, and the Society's discussions were chiefly of a medical nature. The Society was under the patronage of many of the University medical professors including Black, Cullen, Hope and Gregory, and they and other distinguished academic and scientific figures were elected as Honorary members of the Society. A further boost to the Society's status was achieved in 1788 when it obtained a Royal Charter. After 1827, the Society began to broaden its interests to more general scientific and natural history subjects, and gradually attracted more resident members than its previous rapid turn-over of medical students.

Objects

The cultivation of the natural and physical sciences.

Membership

Began with eighteen members, but grew rapidly with accession of members from other medical and natural history societies. Had 133 Resident Fellows in 1878, but the overall number of Fellows around the world has always been much greater: 440 Fellows in 1780; 1300 in 1830; 1600 in 1853.

Meetings

Originally on the fourth Wednesday of every month.

Publications

Laws of the Royal Physical Society (Edinburgh, 1819).
Proceedings of the Royal Physical Society published regularly after first volume in 1858.

Records

Minute books held by Royal Physical Society, Edinburgh.
Twenty-eight volumes of transcripts, containing essays read between 1783/4–1827/8 in Special Collections, Edinburgh University Library.

Secondary References

Finlayson (1956–8), 7–8.
Hume (1853), 172–3.
McElroy (1952), 302, 304–8, 311.
McElroy (1969), 136–8.
Med.Dir., passim.
Year-Book, passim.

52. Fife Medico-Chirurgical Society* (1825–40>)

History

The Society had wide-ranging plans for the educational and professional needs of the medical community in Fife, and by 1827 had assembled a library of 130 medical volumes. In October 1828, the Secretary of the Society, Robert Wisemann, a Cupar surgeon, sent a circular to all medical practitioners in Fife, calling attention to the existence of the Society. Also enclosed was a copy of a table of medical charges for the area drawn up by the Society which has not survived. Further copies of the fee schedules were offered to individual practitioners at a rate of ten shillings per hundred. The Circular also referred to a new class of membership, local corresponding members, devised by the Society after its formation. This recognised the difficulty those living elsewhere in the area had travelling to the meetings in Cupar. In addition, the circular mentioned the possibility of holding an annual meeting of the Society elsewhere in the region. Although no definite date of cessation has been identified, it is possible that the failure to attract medical practitioners from outside the immediate environs of Cupar as members, caused the Society to fail. *The Society changed its title to the Fife Medico-Chirurgical Association sometime before 1840.

Objects

'... to promote Medical Science, and a friendly discourse among the Faculty in Fife; to establish a Library and Museum; to read Dissertations on Medical subjects periodically...'. (Laws of the Fife Medico-Chirurgical Society, 1827)

Membership

Open to qualified medical practitioners in Fife. Entrance fee was one guinea, plus a further guinea annually. The Society had thirteen members in 1827.

Meetings

Originally quarterly in Cupar on the first Friday in January, April, July and October, at 1 p.m.. By 1840, meetings were annual, in October.

Publications

Laws of the Fife Medico-Chirurgical Society (Cupar, 1827).

Records

N.L. The printed Laws of the Society, including a catalogue of the Society's Library, and a printed circular notifying the local profession of the Society's existence, are in the National Library of Scotland, Edinburgh.

Secondary References

Ed.Al. (Fife suppl.) (1840), 19.
EMSJ 25 (1826), 241.

53. Fifeshire Colliery Surgeons' Association (<1911–16>)

History

This Association held a joint meeting in Glasgow in July 1911 with the Scottish Midland and Western Medical Association (115), and colliery surgeons from elsewhere in Scotland, to consider the future position of colliery and works surgeons during the discussions of the implications of the National Insurance Bill 1911. As a result of this meeting a joint committee was set up to press the government on the issue of colliery medical practice. Lloyd George, the Chancellor of the Exchequer, refused by letter to meet a deputation from the committee in London, but stated he was quite aware of the difficulties of colliery doctors. Subsequently, an Executive Committee of Scottish Colliery and Public Works Surgeons was established, and continued to protect the interests of colliery and works doctors until at least 1916. The date of cessation of the Fifeshire Colliery Surgeons' Association is unknown.

Objects

To represent the interests of medical practitioners employed as Colliery Surgeons in Fife.

Membership

Open to medical practitioners employed at collieries in the region.

Meetings

F.U.

Publications

N.I.

Records

N.L.

Secondary References

N.I. See Scottish Midland and Western Medical Association, Minute Book, 13 July 1911, and *passim.*

54. Fifeshire Medical Association* (1882–1932)

History

*The Association also went by the name of the Fife Medical Association. At the inaugural meeting of the Association in the Royal Hotel, Cupar, it was decided to give emphasis to social and professional medical interests. Papers delivered before the Association were to be short, and informal discussions of case work were to be preferred. An annual address by the president on a medical or social issue was decided upon, and meetings were to be succeeded by a hearty dinner. In 1885, the subject of the Presidential address, delivered by Robert Spence, a local Parochial Medical officer and Admiralty surgeon in Burntisland, considered the position of Medical Officers of Health in Scotland, and called for the establishment of a centralised Department of Public Health. In 1902, there was some doubt over the future of the Association in the wake of the establishment of a Fife branch of the British Medical Association. But the strong support for the role it played in providing a social forum for local professional matters ensured its survival for a further three decades. The strength of local professional activity at this time is further witnessed by the existence of a Dunfermline and West Fife Medical Association, although nothing more is known of this body, other than its Secretary in 1902 was David Rorie (17).

Objects

To further social interaction and advance the professional interests of medical practitioners in the area.

Membership

The Society was founded with a membership of forty-seven out of sixty medical practitioners residing in Fife.

Meetings

Held in rotation in May and September in Cupar, Kirkcaldy, St. Andrews and Dunfermline.

Publications

N.I.

Records

N.L.

Secondary References

BMJ 1 (1895), 1009.
EMJ 28/1 (1882), 472–6; 31/1 (1885), 246–50; 13 (New series) (1903), 478–9 and *passim.*
Year-Book (1884), 156 and *passim.*

55. Forfar Phrenological Assocation (1835–6>) [L]

History

The Society appears to have played a significant role in intellectual circles in Forfar. Three of the local medical practitioners were members; while Lord Douglas Gordon Hallyburton, MP for Forfarshire from 1831–41, was Honorary President of the Society, and donated a number of casts of heads to its museum (the society also had a small library of phrenological works). The Town-clerk, William Hunter, was President of the Society.

Objects

To advance Phrenological Science.

Membership

Forty two members in 1836. Entrance fee was two shillings and sixpence, plus a further shilling per quarter.

Meetings

Fortnightly, plus additional extraordinary meetings.

Publications

N.I.

Records

N.L.

Secondary References

Cooter (1989), 135, 157–8, 176.
Cottrell Watson (1836), 133–4.

56. Forfarshire Medical Assocation (1858–extant)

History

The Association was formed as a direct result of the passage of the Medical Act of 1858, and sought to protect the professional interests of local medical practitioners. It met annually to hear an address from the President on a medical or medico-professional matter, plus occasional other papers, discussion of which was followed by a dinner in a hotel, to which eminent Scottish medical guests were often invited. In 1864, the Association published its own table of medical fees for the district, based on reports of current rates of fees gathered from the local Secretaries of the Association, and also on information on fees charged elsewhere in Scotland, derived from existing fees tables from nine medical societies. In 1880, the annual meeting discussed the Vaccination Bill then before parliament, which was opposed on the grounds that it allowed for parents to opt out of compulsory vaccination against smallpox for their children on the payment of a fee. The Association drew up a petition to voice its opposition to this proposed piece of legislation. The following year, the question of hygiene in infectious fevers was the subject of the Presidential address delivered by Andrew Key, (formerly Surgeon at Arbroath Infirmary), and this was followed by the results of a committee set up to consider the relative lengths of quarantine for a variety of infectious diseases, in an attempt to promote uniformity of practice among its members in the management of infectious fevers. Although meetings were held on an annual basis, local branches met independently in Arbroath, Brechin, Forfar and Montrose, with separate branch secretaries for these towns elected at the AGM. In 1893, the Association admitted female medical practitioners, one of the first medical societies in Scotland to make this decision. In 1911, the Association communicated with the Dundee Branch of the British Medical Association, to express itself fully in support of the national Association's actions in protest against the Government's introduction introduction of National Health Insurance.

Objects

'Formed to assist the working of the New Medical Act, and to take a general supervision of medical affairs in the county of Forfar'. (*Medical Directory*, 1861, 827)

Membership

Open to qualified practitioners in the area. The Association was formed with 23 original members, it had 30 members in 1862, and 119 members in 1908, and 179 members in 1928. The original annual subscription was two shillings and sixpence. In 1923, the subscription was raised from five shillings to seven shillings and sixpence.

Meetings

Annually in July. Met in rotation in Dundee, Arbroath, Montrose, Brechin and Forfar.

Publications

Annual Report of the Forfarshire Medical Association (Dundee, 1898–1927).
Rules of the Forfarshire Medical Association (Dundee, 1913).
Transactions of the Forfarshire Medical Association (Edinburgh, 1924).

Records

Minute books held by Forfarshire Medical Association. Other printed records including Membership lists, 1858–1908, and reports of annual meetings 1898–1928, in Archive Department, Dundee University Library.

Secondary References

Blair (1990), 61.
BMJ 2 (1895), 99.
EMJ 8 (1862–3), 295; (9 (1863–4), 287–8; 26/1 (1880), 183–5; 32/1 (1886), 380, and *passim.*
Checkland (1980), 187.
Med.Dir,. passim.
Year-Book (1885), 217 and *passim.*

57. Garioch and Northern Medical Association (1854–1925)

History

The Association had a strong interest in medical science and medical politics for the first twenty-five years of its history, but after 1879 no more medical papers were heard. Medical politics continued to excite debate at meetings, as in 1888 when controversy over competition between members of the Association over local appointments as Parochial Board Medical Officers led to acrimonious discussions, and in 1912 when the implications of the National Insurance Act were the subject of conversation. The Association also maintained its representation at the annual meetings of the North of Scotland Medical Association (100), throughout its history. Despite periodic interest in wider medical issues, the main purpose of the Garioch Association in the later part of the nineteenth century until its demise in 1925 was chiefly social, and the business part of each meeting was followed by a dinner.

Objects

The original objects of the Association were to hear papers on medical science, and to discuss the nature and treatment of interesting cases.

Membership

The Association reached a maximum membership of fifty three in 1904, and average membership during its history was thirty three. Membership was open to practitioners practising outside as well as inside the Garioch district.

Meetings

Twice a year, on the first Friday, of May and the last Friday of September. These meetings were later changed to Saturdays. The September meeting represented the AGM and was held in Inverurie.

Publications

Table of Fees of the Garioch and Northern Medical Association (Inverurie, 1863).

Records

Minute books and other papers in Manuscripts Collection, Aberdeen University Library.

Secondary References

Aberdeen Journal, 3 May 1854.

Gordon 'Garioch and Northern Medical Association' ch. in Milne (1989), reprinted from an article of the same name in *Aberdeen Postgraduate Medical Bulletin* (1970), 19–23.

Med.Dir,. passim.

Year-Book (1884), 157 and *passim*.

58. Glasgow and West of Scotland Association of Registered Medical Women* (1904– extant)

History

The Association was formed to further the position of female medical practitioners in the West of Scotland, and discussions were originally limited to professional and ethical matters. No papers on medical topics were read. It was for this reason that the Association was refused affiliation with the London Association of Registered Medical Women in January 1905, when the Glasgow Association's Secretary, Louise McIlroy, former House Surgeon at the Samaritan Hospital and at Glasgow Royal Infirmary, and subsequently Assistant Gynaecological Surgeon at Glasgow Royal Infirmary (71), wrote to the London Secretary enquiring about affiliation in order for Glasgow members to use the London Association's library and facilities when in the capital. This position had altered by 1916, when the Glasgow Association joined with twenty three other local associations of registered medical women from around the country to establish the Medical Women's Federation. *In 1918, the Glasgow Association changed its name to the Scottish Western Association of the Medical Women's Federation. In 1919, the newly created Western and Eastern (111) Scottish branches of the MWF decided to meet together under the name of the Scottish Union of Medical Women (125) for the purpose of considering issues affecting the whole of the female Scottish medical profession; these joint meetings continued until 1932.

Objects

'To form a bond of union among the women in practice in Glasgow and the West of Scotland; to look after the interests of medical women generally...' (Session card 1905–6, Glasgow and West of Scotland Association of Registered Medical Women)

Membership

Twenty nine members in 1905. Annual subscription was two shillings and sixpence.

Meetings

The Glasgow Association met three times annually, with meetings held in members' houses. The Western Association now meets on a monthly basis from October to June.

Publications

N.I.

Records

Records to 1942 held by the Honorary Secretary, Scottish Western Association of the Medical Women's Federation. Correspondence and membership card of Glasgow Association in Medical Women's Federation papers (SA/MWF c. 76; c.77–9) in Contemporary Archives, Wellcome Institute Library, London.

Secondary References
N.I.

59. Glasgow and West of Scotland Medical Association (1866–1944*)

History

The Association is unique in terms of Scottish medical societies in that it was established with the avowed purpose of guaranteeing the future of the *Glasgow Medical Journal*, which had gone through a series of financial difficulties since its inception in 1828. The establishment of the Association and its guarantee of financial backing enabled the *Journal* to be placed on a sound footing. *In 1944, the Association merged with the Royal Medico-Chirurgical Society of Glasgow (104), and this Society, in conjunction with the Scottish Society for Experimental Medicine (122), continues to fund the publication of the *Scottish Medical Journal*.

Objects

'... [The] principal object shall be the promotion of Medical Science by the publication of a journal to be called the *Glasgow Medical Journal*.' (Printed Regulations of the Glasgow and West of Scotland Medical Association, 1875)

Membership

Two classes of membership, guaranteeing and non-guaranteeing, the former paid £5 and became the managing body of the *Journal*. In addition, all members paid an annual subscription of twelve shillings, subsequently raised to £1. In June 1868 the Association had 115 subscribing members, this had risen to 254 by August of that year. In 1884, the membership is given as 'under 500'.

Meetings

Annual meeting in October, later changed to January.

Publications

Glasgow Medical Journal, 1868–1944.
Printed Regulations of the Glasgow and West of Scotland Medical Association (Glasgow, 1875).

Records

Minute books and Treasurer's accounts in the Royal College of Physicians and Surgeons, Glasgow.

Secondary References
EMJ 16 (1870–71), 672.
GMJ 109 (1928), 86–7, and *passim*.
Med.Dir,. passim.
Year-Book (1884), 158 and *passim*.

60. Glasgow Curative Mesmeric Association (1861–2?) [L]

History

Weekly meetings of the Association were held '... for the purpose of receiving and disposing of applications for treatment; for reporting cases of alleviation and cure, and for mutual encouragement and advice'. The Glasgow Association was affiliated to the Scottish Curative Mesmeric Association (124), based in Edinburgh. According to the Association's *First Annual Report* over 300 patients had been treated mesmerically by members of the Association. William Naismith (former House Surgeon at Glasgow Royal Infirmary), was a member of the Association's acting committee in 1862. The Association rented a hall for its meetings, paid for by the subscriptions of members and supporters of mesmerism, and had begun the process of compiling a library of works on mesmerism, phrenology and general medical science by the end of its first year of existence.

Objects

'1. To apply Mesmerism to the Cure and Alleviation of Disease; and 2. To encourage its use by all classes in the community.' (Consitution of the Glasgow Curative Mesmeric Association, 1862)

Membership

Sixteen members in 1862.

Meetings

Weekly on Fridays at 8 p.m. in the Mesmeric Hall, Wilson Street.

Publications

First Annual Report of the Glasgow Curative Mesmeric Association (Glasgow, 1862).

Records

N.L. Report of the Association in National Library of Scotland, Edinburgh.

Secondary References

Cooter (1989), 182.

61. Glasgow Eastern Medical Society (1893–1933*)

History

The Eastern Medical Society had a significant scientific and professional output from its earliest days. In an 1896 report of a meeting on Rheumatoid Arthritis addressed by a guest speaker from Buxton, the *Lancet* remarked upon the Society's vitality and enterprise. In professional matters too, the Society was active. The previous year, the *BMJ* reported on the Society's proposals for: reform of the General Medical Council; improved contracts for Parochial Medical Officers, and for doctors employed by friendly societies and clubs; and the regulation of dispensary treatment. Between 1900 and 1901, representatives of the Society formed a conjoint committee with the Glasgow Southern Medical Society (80) and the Glasgow and West of Scotland branch of the BMA to campaign against the prosecution of West of Scotland practitioners by the Pharmaceutical Association of Great Britain for employing unqualified medical dispensers in their surgeries. Reports of the Society's meetings were given in the *GMJ* for much of its history. *The Society was revived between 1968 and 1982.

Objects

To further medical science and promote the interests of the profession.

Membership

No details of size or cost of membership. The Society elected six office bearers, six council members and two auditors annually.

Meetings

Initially on the second Wednesday of each month at 9 p.m. in the Hall of Sydney Place United Presbyterian Church, Duke Street, later meetings were held fortnightly in the same location.

Publications

N.I.

Records

Records of Conjoint Committee of the Eastern and Southern Glasgow Medical Societies and the local BMA branch, 1900–1, are held in the Library, Victoria Infirmary, Glasgow.

Secondary References
BMJ 2 (1895), 1072.
GMJ 58 (1902), 379–82 and *passim.*
Lancet 1 (1896), 590.
Med.Dir., *passim.*
Year-Book, (1895), 238 and *passim.*

62. Glasgow Faculty of Medicine (1825–1904)

History

This organisation was formed out of irritation felt by sections of the profession in Glasgow with the high fees charged by the Faculty of Physicians and Surgeons to obtain the Licence required for legal practice in the City and surrounding area. This, plus the large levy required to join the compulsory Widow's Fund made for dissatisfaction among the rank and file of the profession. It is clear from its title, and the setting up of a (more affordable) Widow's Fund, that the Faculty of Medicine (FM) was formed as a rival institution to the Faculty of Physicians and Surgeons (FPSG). Although it could not challenge the Licensing powers of the latter body, the fact that the FM was listed in the Western Supplement of the *Edinburgh Almanac* for 1835 alongside the FPSG and the Faculty of Procurators, and that these three organisations listed separately from other literary and scientific societies, demonstrates the aspirations of its members to challenge the position of the FPSG.

In 1828, a free vaccination dispensary was instituted by the Faculty of Medicine, and this service continued for sixty years. The FM's service was provided in the building of a charitable medical organisation which for a time also offered free vaccination to the city's population, the 'Glasgow Cow Pock Institution', and the Hall came to be known as 'Cow Pock Hall'. The reading of medical papers was introduced into the Faculty's activities after a short time, and reports of these appeared in the *Glasgow Medical Examiner* in the course of 1831–2. Towards the end of its history, and perhaps due to the proliferation of medical societies in the city, the Faculty became restricted to a medical reading club. The FM was referred to by the local profession as the 'wee Faculty'.

Objects

'Originated for the purpose of establishing a Medical Library, a free Vaccine Institution, and for other Medical Purposes.' (*Medical Directory* (1853), 785)

Membership

Open to qualified medical practitioners in Glasgow. Fees were two guineas annually.

Meetings

On the first Friday of each month at 5 p.m. in 'Cow Pock Hall', St. Andrew's Square, later meetings were held in the city's Eye Infirmary.

Publications

N.I.

Records

Minute books and other records are held in the Library of the Royal College of Physicians, Glasgow.

Secondary References
Duncan (1896), 195–6.
Glasgow Medical Examiner (1831–1832), *passim.*
GMJ 96 (1920), 49.
Ed.Al. (*Glasgow suppl.*), *passim.*

Med.Dir,. passim.
Year-Book (1891), 210 and *passim.*

63. Glasgow Medical Club (1798–1814?)

History

The Glasgow Medical Club was a social club for the professional medical elite in the city, akin to those which proliferated in eighteenth-century Edinburgh. Its members were leading figures in the Faculty of Physicians and Surgeons of Glasgow, and included the Professor of Medicine at Glasgow University, Robert Freer. He, and other members of the Club were among the original directors of the recently-established Glasgow Royal Infirmary (1794). James Jeffray, Professor of Anatomy at Glasgow University was also a member. The Club was a tight-knit body and applicants for membership were excluded if there was one negative among those voting. Young members of the medical profession were not recruited to its ranks and the Club came to an abrupt end after approximately fifteen years.

Objects

To cement the bonds of friendship among members of the profession in the city.

Membership

Formed with twelve members.

Meetings

Monthly in a local tavern at 4 p.m.

Publications

N.I.

Records

N.L.

Secondary References

Duncan (1896), 197.
Strang (1864), 241–2; 247–51.

64. Glasgow Medical Lunch Club (1921–22>)

History

The first meeting of the Club, formed under the auspices of the Glasgow Eastern Division of the BMA, was held in Ferguson and Forrester's Restaurant in the city's Buchanan Street, and was attended by over forty medical practitioners. John Glaister (then Regius Professor of Forensic Medicine and Public Health at the University of Glasgow) (65) was the Club's first Guest speaker, and spoke of the useful purpose such a Club could serve in medical matters, particularly as a means of communication regarding municipal health problems and state projects. The Club was placed on a permanent footing in 1922 with the election of three office-bearers and a committee of nine, including Osborne Henry Mavor, a former House Surgeon at Glasgow Royal Infirmary (77), perhaps better known under his pseudonym as the playwright James Bridie. The ultimate fate of the Club is not known.

Objects

To hold a lunch for medical practitioners at which an invited guest medical speaker would address the company.

Membership

Open to all medical practitioners in Glasgow and its neighbourhood.

Meetings
Held every two months.
Publications
N.I.
Records
N.L.
Secondary References
GMJ 98 (1922), 47–8; 344, and *passim.*

65. Glasgow Medical Missionary Society (1868–1975>) [L]
History
Like other medical mission societies, the Glasgow Society originally had a dual purpose: to train medical men for mission work overseas, and to provide free medical aid for the poor in the city. A dispensary was established in the City, and the hope was to encourage medical students towards missionary work through care of the poor in the city. The provision of medical aid for the Glasgow poor soon became the paramount intention of the Society. The staff of the dispensary remained small, however, and aid from the qualified medical profession was financial, rather than practical. In 1890, the Society maintained two dispensaries, each under the charge of a qualified medical superintendent, and 40,000 consultations were heard. Despite expansion in state health provision, it is clear that the Society still had a role to play in to the twentieth century. At its sixtieth annual meeting in 1928, with the Society over £250 in debt, Professor John Glaister (64) referred to the fact that no person receiving National Health Insurance or who was in receipt of Parish Relief was entitled to benefit from the Mission, suggesting that claims on the dispensary services were outstripping their provision.

Objects
For the benefit of those who require, but are not able to pay for a Doctor, and are not provided for by the Parish.

Membership
Open to members of the profession, medical students, and other interested individuals.

Meetings
Held an annual business meeting.

Publications
Glasgow Medical Missionary Society Annual Reports (1868–?).

Records
N.L.

Secondary References
BMJ 2 (1890), 1445.
Checkland (1980), 82–4.
Ed.Al. (Western Suppl.), (1872), 84, *passim.*
GMJ 98 (1922), 53; 109 (1928), 61–2, *passim.*
Glasgow Post Office Directory (1952/3), 266, *passim.*

66. Glasgow Medical Society (1814–66*)
History
In its first years, members of the Society were obliged to deliver papers in rotation, and

failure to do so was met by a fine. There were also fines for lateness and for failure to attend meetings. These regulations suggest the Society was intent in creating a serious atmosphere for the pursuit of medical science, but they also placed a heavy burden on the members of the Society, which remained relatively small in number, and there was a high turn-over in membership. Despite its avowed purpose to further medical science, there were papers on other issues, including medical ethics and education. The essays serve as a reflection of the current medical developments with papers delivered on subjects as the benefits of ether and chloroform as anaesthetic agents in 1847 and 1848 respectively. *The Society amalgamated with the still flourishing (Royal) Medico-Chirurgical Society of Glasgow (105) in 1866. Although not rivals, with many local practitioners members of both, it was felt by conjoint committees of the Societies' that union would increase their influence and prosperity, and save on any duplication of activities that may have previously occurred. The final meeting of the Glasgow Medical Society was held in March 1866.

Objects

'... the prosecution of Medical Science'. (Society Minutes, 27 October 1814)

Membership

Founded with eight members, had twenty members in 1815. Entrance fee was one guinea.

Meetings

On the first and third Tuesdays of each month from October to May in the Hall of the Faculty of Physicians and Surgeons, Glasgow.

Publications

N.I.

Records

Minute books and thirty-one bound volumes of essays delivered before the Society between 1814–45 are held in the Library of the Royal College of Physicians and Surgeons, Glasgow.

Secondary References

Dow and Calman (1989), 5–29.
Walker Downie (1908), 2–39.
Duncan (1896), 187–92.
Power (1939), 63–77.
See also *Ed. Al. (Glasgow Suppl.)* and *Med.Dir., passim.*

67. Glasgow Medico-Chirurgical Society* (1820–32)

History

*This relatively short-lived Society is not to be confused with the (Royal) Medico-Chirurgical Society of Glasgow (104), which is still in existence. The Society originated in a meeting of three local medical practitioners, and the Society first met in members houses, although it later met in 'Cow Pock Hall', St. Andrews Square, the meeting place of the Glasgow Faculty of Medicine (64). The Society's regulations provided for the compulsory reading of papers, and employed the use of fines for members who failed to participate, and these factors may have had some bearing on the size and brevity of the Society's existence.

Objects

The Society met '... for the purpose of writing and discussing medical subjects'. (Society minutes, 13 June 1820)

Membership

A small society, with nine members in 1822. Total membership between 1820–32 was twenty-one.

Meetings

Initially weekly on Thursdays at 8 p.m., later meetings were held fortnightly.

Publications

N.I.

Records

Minute book in the Royal College of Physicians and Surgeons, Glasgow.

Secondary References

Dow (1989), 301.
Walker Downie (1908), 40–1.
Ed.Al. (Glasgow suppl.), passim.
GMJ 55 (1899), 333–5.
Power (1939), 70.

68. Glasgow Microscopical Society (1886–1931*) [L]

History

Medical and biological papers using microscopic sections as illustrations were delivered before the Society. In addition, demonstrations of microscope technology were given by Society members. Most contributions were made by medical practitioners. The Society was under the Presidency of James Rankin of the Zoological laboratory, Glasgow University from 1897–1901, the years in which it featured in the *Year-Book of Scientific and Literary Societies.* *The Society was incorporated into the Glasgow and Andersonian Natural History and Microscopical Society in 1931.

Objects

To further microscopic science through papers illustrated by lantern slides and by demonstrations of microscopic sections.

Membership

Open to all with an interest in microscopic research.

Meetings

Monthly on the third Tuesday of each month, from September to April.

Publications

N.I.

Records

N.L.

Secondary References

Glasgow Post Office Directory 1952/3, 2129.
Lancet 1 (1896), 811; 1175.
Nuttall, 'Early Scottish Microscopes' (1981), 199–200.
Year-Book (1897), 127 and *passim.*

69. Glasgow North Western Medical Society (1872–6?)

History

This Society appears to have been intended to serve the interests of local general practitioners, since none of its office-bearers held hospital or teaching appointments in the city. There are no details available on papers read or discussions held by members of the Society.

Objects

To further the professional interests of local practitioners through regular meetings in a social atmosphere.

Membership

Open to qualified practitioners in the north west of the city.

Meetings

Fortnightly on Thursdays at 8.30 p.m. from October to May in a hotel in the centre of Glasgow.

Publications

N.I.

Records

N.L.

Secondary References

Med.Dir,. (1875–6).

70. Glasgow Northern Medical Society (1902–53)

History

The Glasgow Northern Medical Society was established to provide a professional focus for practitioners located in the north of the city (including the city centre). In 1912, a discussion on the reform of the General Medical Council, to increase the number of directly-elected members, and at the same time increase the voice of the rank and file of the profession, led to the establishment of a committee to draw a memorial on the issue and to canvass the opinions of other local medical societies on the issue. No further details of this project are known, although the Society was soon to be one of many societies whose proceedings were halted for the duration of the First World War, as medical personnel joined the armed forces, and those remaining at home were faced with an increase in their work load. Regular meetings of the Society were resumed in September 1919. In 1925 a special meeting was convened to discuss the introduction of a proposed scale of minimum fees. During the 1920s the Society held annual excursions and a golf competiton for members. Reports of Society meetings and annual lists of the Society's office-bearers were printed in the *GMJ*.

Objects

To hear papers on medical and collateral subjects; to promote social relationships between members; and to offer advice on matters affecting the interests of the profession.

Membership

Established with twenty-one members in 1902. In 1924, they had 113 members. Annual subscription was five shillings.

Meetings

On the first Tuesday of each month at 8.30 p.m., at the Glasgow Royal Philosophical Society's Hall, October–May. Annual meeting held in May.

Publications

Constitution of Glasgow Northern Medical Society (Glasgow, 1903).

Records

Minute books held in the Library of the Royal College of Physicians, Glasgow.

Secondary References
GMJ 75 (1912), 140–1; 98 (1922), 363 and *passim*.
Lancet 2 (1902), 1093.
Med.Dir,. passim.
Year-Book (1913), 370 and *passim*.

71. Glasgow Obstetrical and Gynaecological Society (1885–extant)

History

This Society has been open to both general practitioners and specialists from its inception. In 1893 it became one of the first Scottish medical societies to admit female practitioners, and Louise McIlroy (58), was elected Vice-President for the 1912–13 session. In the years before the outbreak of the First World War the Society held well-attended conjoint meetings with both the Edinburgh Obstetrical Society (42) and the North of England Obstetrical and Gynaecological Society. The Glasgow Obstetrical and Gynaecological Society did not meet between 1914 and 1921 due to the wartime situation, and between 1921–4 it met only periodically. In 1924, the Society was reconstituted to include more informal, clinical meetings at Glasgow Royal Maternity Hospital, a move which improved attendances and gave new impetus to the Society, which celebrated its centenary in 1985.

Objects

'The promotion of science and art in connection with midwifery and the diseases of women and children.' (Society minutes, June 17 1885)

Membership

Fellowship open to all qualified practitioners on nomination of three Fellows, and a two-thirds majority in a ballot of Fellows present. Annual subscription was originally five shillings a year. Society had eighty-five fellows in 1885.

Meetings

On the fourth Wednesday of each month, from October to June, at 8 p.m. in the Hall of the Faculty of Physicians and Surgeons, Glasgow.

Publications

Transactions of the Glasgow Obstetrical and Gynaecological Society published from 1889.

Records

Surviving minute books in the Library of the Royal College of Physicians and Surgeons of Glasgow.

Secondary References

Christie (1888), 185.
Dow (1989), 47–48.
EMJ 35/1 (1885), 197 and *passim*.
GMJ 41 (1885) and *passim*.
Glasgow News, 21 May 1885.
SMJ 33 (1988), 378–80.
See also *Med.Dir.* and *Year-Book, passim*.

72. Glasgow Odontological Society (1902–58>)

History

Although the Diploma in Dental Surgery was offered at Anderson's College after 1879, there was no local representative organisation in the city beyond the short-lived Society of Licentiates in Dental Surgery (126). Before the institution of the Glasgow

Odintological Society qualified dental surgeons in the city were solely represented by the West of Scotland Branch of the British Dental Association. In 1908, the Society established an annual prize for senior dental students to be judged on their practical work. After 1920, the Society held annual joint meetings with the Odonto-Chirurgical Society of Scotland and the Dundee Dental Club which were held in rotation in Edinburgh, Glasgow and Dundee.

Objects

To promote professional interests and social relationships between qualified dental surgeons.

Membership

Open to all qualified dental practitioners in Glasgow.

Meetings

F.U.

Publications

N.I.

Records

N.L.

Secondary References

British Journal of Dental Science, passim.
Brown Henderson (1960), 2.
Menzies Campbell (1958), 245.
Year-Book (1925), 395 and *passim.*

73. Glasgow Pathological Society* (1850–4)

History

*This society had no link with the later Glasgow Pathological and Clinical Society (74). The Pathological Society met in Glasgow Royal Infirmary, and the Society's Secretary, J.C. Steele was Superintendent at the Infirmary. In 1854, with the Society obviously ailing, a Council member of the Pathological Society, J. B. Cowan, who was also a member of the Glasgow Medical Society (66), raised the matter of amalgamation with the older Society, but his proposal was not taken up and the Society ended shortly thereafter.

Objects

To further the study of pathology, through discussion and examination of specimens.

Membership

No specific details. The Society had eight office-bearers and council members in 1851.

Meetings

F.U.

Publications

N.I.

Records

N.L.

Secondary References

Dow (1989), 27.
Walker Downie (1908), 38.
Duncan (1896), 196–7.
Ed.Al. (Western suppl.) (1851), 74.

74. Glasgow Pathological and Clinical Society (1873–1907*)

History

Formed under the Presidency of William Tennant Gairdner, then Professor of Pathology at Glasgow University (31, 39, 41, 47, 50), and with twenty-one founder members, the Society was known as the Pathological Society during its first session, and meetings were held at the City's Lying-in Hospital in Wellington street. In the course of the second session, the more clinical aspects of the Society's discussion were recognised and the name of the Society was altered to the Pathological and Clinical Society. From 1877, the Society met in the Hall of the Faculty of Physicians and Surgeons. In 1903, female medical practitioners were admitted to the Society. *The Society was amalgamated with the Royal Medico-Chirurgical Society of Glasgow (104) in 1907.

Objects

The exhibition and study of patients, preparations, drawings and instruments.

Membership

The number of members was limited, at first to thirty, and later to forty, to ensure the Society was a working, active group. At the time of its amlagamation with the (Royal) Medico-Chirurgical Society of Glasgow the Society had seventy three memebrs.

Meetings

Monthly from October to May on the second Tuesday of each month at 8 p.m.

Publications

Transactions of the Glasgow Pathological and Clinical Society published bi-annually in eleven volumes between 1884 and 1908.

Records

Minute books, membership lists and other MS material in the Library of the Royal College of Physicians and Surgeons, Glasgow.

Secondary References

Christie (1888), 184.
Walker Downie (1908), 77–88.
Duncan (1896), 197.
Kerr, 'Royal Medico-Chirurgical Society of Glasgow' (1938), 94.
Power (1939), 75–6.
See also *BMJ*, *Ed.Al.* (Western Suppl.), *GMJ*, *Med.Dir.* and *Year-Book, passim.*

75. Glasgow Phrenological Society (1829–45) [L]

History

Although not formally constituted as a Society until 1829, interest in phrenological science in Glasgow, particularly among the medical profession, was strong throughout the 1820s. Two series of public lectures on phrenology were delivered in Glasgow in this decade by William Weir, physician at Glasgow Royal Infirmary, and Robert Hunter, Professor of Anatomy at Anderson's University, later Professor of Anatomy and Surgery at Portland Street Medical School (86). Weir also lectured to medical students on phrenology in 1821, as he was to do less successfully, twenty years later. Both Weir and Hunter were future Presidents of the Faculty of Physicians and Surgeons, Glasgow. In 1835, Weir was Vice-President of the Phrenological Society, and in the following year the Society set up its own library and museum. In 1845/6, Weir began a series of lectures on phrenology to medical students at Anderson's University, but these were soon discontinued due to lack of interest among the students, and indeed, by the mid-1840s scientific interest in phrenology was in decline.

Objects

To advance the science of phrenology.

Membership

Forty-nine members in 1836. Entrance fee was ten shillings and sixpence, with an annual subscription of four shillings.

Meetings

Fortnightly.

Publications

Phrenological Almanack (1842–6).

Records

N.L. See Letter-book of Edinburgh Phrenological Society Nov. 24 1824 in Special Collections, Edinburgh University Library, for reference to phrenological meetings in Glasgow. See also Anderson's Institution Minute Book and Attendance Book of Popular Evening Classes, Strathclyde University Archives Department, for reference to the history of the Chair of Phrenology at the University 1845–7, and to a meeting of Glasgow Phrenological Society in 1837, respectively.

Secondary References

Cooter (1984), 90, 287, 298.
Cooter (1989), 175, 191, 341, 351.
Ed.Al. (Western suppl.) (1835), 51 and *passim.*
Phrenological Almanack, passim.
Cottrell Watson (1836), 135–8.

76. Glasgow Royal Infirmary Medical Society (1881–94)

History

The Society was one of a number of groups set up to cater for the educational and social needs of medical staff in Scottish hospitals.

Objects

To promote the educational and social interaction between members of the medical staff of Glasgow Royal Infirmary.

Membership

Open to members of staff at Glasgow Royal Infirmary.

Meetings

F.U.

Publications

N.I.

Records

Minute book in the Library of the Royal College of Physicians and Surgeons, Glasgow.

Secondary References

N.I.

77. Glasgow Royal Infirmary Club (1897–1922>)

History

This was a social club open to current and former resident medical staff members of Glasgow Royal Infirmary, including female residents, and featured many of the leading members of the profession in the West of Scotland in the early twentieth century. In 1922, when the Club held its twenty-fifth annual dinner, Osborne Henry Mavor (64) was Joint-Secretary. It is probable that the Club had its origins in the Glasgow Royal Infirmary Medical Society (76), which ceased shortly before the Club came into being, although no information on this matter has been located.

Objects

To foster social relations between resident staff members.

Membership

Open to past and present residents of Glasgow Royal Infirmary. 258 members in 1913.

Meetings

Annual dinner and business meeting on the second Friday of March.

Publications

N.I.

Records

N.L.

Secondary References

Wallace Anderson (1916), i, 49.
GMJ 75 (1911), 363–4; 79 (1913), 281; 98 (1922), 237–8.
Lancet 1 (1908), 461.

78. Glasgow Southern Medical Society (1844–extant)

History

The Southern Medical Society was established by a small group of general practitioners, and in its early years met in the homes of its members. At a meeting of the Society in 1878, Ebenezeer Duncan, a local general practitioner and Surgeon at the Glasgow Deaf and Dumb Institute, first proposed the construction of a hospital to serve the growing population on the city's south side. The Society took up this call, and formed a committee of investigation into the requirements of a hospital for the area. The Society was also later represented on the committee which gathered funds to support the construction of the Victoria Infirmary. In recognition of the role played by the Southern Medical Society in the campaign for the construction of the Victoria Infirmary, it was represented by a member of the Society on the hospital's governing body. The nominated governor made an annual report on the Infirmary's activities to the Society.

   Although open to all ranks of male medical practitioners, the Southern Medical Society maintained its early links with the rank and file of the profession, and in the years 1900–2, was very active in the campaign to defend from prosecution medical practitioners in the West of Scotland who employed unqualified assistants in their dispensaries, or 'shops' as they were then called (see chapter five for more on this campaign). The Society was held in abeyance between 1915 and 1919, and meetings on war medical work characterised the early post-war years. Between 1928 and 1931 the Society held several joint meetings with the Glasgow Southern Women's Medical Society (79), but no women were admitted to the Society until 1979.

Objects

'Mutual improvement in professional knowledge and mutual assistance in professional duties when required.' (Laws of the Society, 1851)

Membership

Open to qualified male medical practitioners. Female practitioners were admitted in 1979.

Meetings

Originally held fortnightly on Thursdays, from October to May.

Publications

Dougall, *Historical Sketch of the Glasgow Southern Medical Society* (Glasgow, 1888).
Laws of the Glasgow Southern Medical Society (Glasgow, 1851), (reprinted eleven times, last occasion, 1980).

Records

Minute books and other MS are held in the Library, Victoria Infirmary, Glasgow

Secondary References

Dow and Slater (1990), *passim.*
Slater, 'Glasgow Southern Medical Society 100 Years Ago' (1988), 24–31.
——, 'Further Centennial Reflections on the Glasgow Southern Medical Society' (1989), 20–7.
——, '1888–1889, the Year of The Victoria Infirmary: from the Minutes of the Glasgow Southern Medical Society' (1990), 22–9.
See also *BMJ, Med.Dir., GMJ, Lancet, Year-Book, passim.*

79. Glasgow Southern Women's Medical Society (<1927–31>)

History

This Society was established to represent the professional interests of female practitioners on the south side of the city. Its origins lay in the continued refusal of the Glasgow Southern Medical Society (78) to admit female practitioners to its ranks. The Southern Women's Society held a number of conjoint meetings with the Southern Medical Society between 1927 and 1931, including clinical meetings in the Victoria Infirmary, medico-political discussions, and the Southern Medical Society's Annual picnic.

Objects

To represent the professional interests of female medical practitioners.

Membership

Open to qualified female practitioners. No details on the size of the Society, six members attended a joint meeting with Southern Medical Society in 1931.

Meetings

F.U.

Publications

N.I.

Records

N.L. See Minutes of Glasgow Southern Medical Society, 28 April 1927; 22 March 1928; 9 May 1929; 8 May 1930; 29 January 1931.

Secondary References

N.L.

80. Glasgow Western Medical Society* (1907–25)

History

The Western Medical Society was set up to provide practitioners in the expanding west-end of Glasgow with a local medical society similar to those already in existence in the east (61); north (70); and south (78) of Glasgow. Medical practitioners from Partick, Hyndland, Whiteinch and Scotstoun, joined the Society, which was formed with six office-bearers, and a council of eight. *In 1908, the Society was renamed the Partick and District Medical Society. In that year the Society appointed a General Debt Collector in an attempt to recover outstanding debts from patients. In October 1910 the first general meeting of the Society's session was devoted to a discussion on the 'Notification of Phthisis', which was opened by Ernest Watt, Medical Officer of Health and Police Surgeon for the Burgh of Partick, and Superintendent of Knightswood Hospital. The Society continued to meet during the course of World War One, and particular emphasis was given to professional salary issues. In November 1918, the Society held a general discussion on the 'present state of the medical profession in Partick'.

Objects

'... to afford its members opportunities of meeting socially, and of formally discussing at regular intervals matters of ethical and educational interest.' (*BMJ* (1908), 711–12)

Membership

The Society had forty eight members in 1917. Annual subscription was five shillings.

Meetings

On the second Thursday of each month at 8.30 p.m. in Partick Burgh Halls.

Publications

N.I.

Records

Minute book in Library Royal College of Physicians, Glasgow.

Secondary References

BMJ 1 (1908), 711–12.
GMJ 75 (1911), 57–8 and *passim*.
See also *Med.Dir.* and *Year-Book, passim*.

81. Govan Medical Society (<1911–27>)

History

Little is known about this Society except in through its relationships to other medical societies. First mention of it appears in the minutes of the council of the Glasgow and West of Scotland Branch of the BMA in 1911, in the course of an oblique reference to the Govan Cottage Nurses Home, but there is no further information supplied. In 1913 and again in 1926, the President of the Society was invited along with other Glasgow medical society presidents to the annual dinner of the Glasgow Southern Medical Society (78). In 1927, during a debate on the admission of female practitioners into the Glasgow Southern, it was mentioned that the Govan Medical Society admitted female practitioners to its ranks.

Objects

No details.

Membership

Open to local male and female medical practitioners.

Meetings

F.U.

Publications

N.I.

Records

N.L. See Glasgow Southern Medical Society Council minute book, 16 October 1913;

minute book, 11 November 1926; 28 April 1927; Glasgow and West of Scotland Branch of the BMA council minute book, 13 October 1911; all held in Library, Glasgow Victoria Infirmary.

Secondary References

N.I.

82. Granton Club (1841–53)

History

The Granton was a dining and social club of exclusive membership. Granton was at this time a small spa town outside Edinburgh, where the social Club's annual excursions were held. Among the eleven founder members who attended the inaugural dinner at the Granton Hotel, were three medical professors of Edinburgh University: Syme, Christison (93) and Traill, the Professors of Clinical Surgery, Materia Medica, and Medical Jurisprudence, respectively. The clubs ties with the University's Medical Faculty are made even more explicit by the fact that the annual dinner of the club was to be held on the first Friday after graduation day at the University.

Objects

To hold an annual dinner and excursion to Granton for its members and invited medical guests.

Membership

By invitation only. The Club had an average of thirteen members during its history, reaching a peak of seventeen in 1845.

Meetings

Held annual dinner.

Publications

N.I.

Records

Minute book in the Library of the Royal College of Physicians, Edinburgh.

Secondary References

N.I.

83. Greenock Faculty of Medicine* (1907–extant)

History

The Faculty, which was a medical society in all but name, continued the trend of professional medical union in the town, following two previous medical societies, the Greenock Medical and Chirurgical Association (84) and the Greenock Medical Society (85). In 1910, Robert Fullerton, Surgeon in the Out-door Department for Diseases of Throat and Nose, Glasgow Royal Infirmary, gave an address as Honorary President of the Greenock Faculty of Medicine, based on his years in practise in Greenock, on the rise of Laryngology and Rhinology as specialities. *Some time during the course of World War One the society's title was changed to the 'Greenock and District Faculty of Medicine'.

Objects

To further the educational, professional and social interests of its members.

Membership

Open to qualified practitioners in Greenock and surrounding areas.

Meetings

Originally on the first Wednesday of the month at 8.30 p.m., from October to April at Greenock Infirmary.

Publications

N.I.

Records

Held by the Greenock and District Faculty of Medicine.

Secondary References

GMJ 75 (1911), 81.
Med.Dir,. passim.
Year-Book (1911), 365 and *passim.*

84. Greenock Medical and Chirurgical Association (1818–51*)

History

The Association possessed a library for the use of its members, and for a time offered a vaccination service to the local population, although this was discontinued by 1831. In 1841, William Turner the President of the Association, reported his attendance at a general meeting of Heritors and Kirk sessions regarding the appointment and salary rates for medical officers to the poor in the district. The Association's activities in this matter were deemed to be rewarded with the appointment of three district surgeons at a salary of £20 a year, with an additional allowance of £5 for medicines. In 1845, the Association held a discussion on a bill to amend the Medical Act which was then before Parliament, and recorded their support for its content. Among the medical discussions held by the Association was one on the treatment of epilepsy in 1846. The following year the lack of sanitary provision and regulation in Greenock was discussed. *In 1850–1 the Association's membership was reduced to just six members, who decided to divide the library collection of over four hundred books between themselves for safe-keeping until the Association could be reconvened on a firmer footing, although there is no record of this taking place.

Objects

'For promoting professional intercourse and improvement'. (*Edinburgh Almanack*, Western suppl. (1828), 544)

Membership

The Association had six members in 1850. Membership fee was one guinea to be paid into the library fund, and two shillings and sixpence for the ordinary fund.

Meetings

On the first Wednesday of the month from November and April.

Publications

Laws and Regulations of Greenock Medical and Chirurgical Association 1820–21 (Greenock, 1821).

Records

Minute book for 1840–51 in the Library of the Royal College of Physicians and Surgeons, Glasgow.

Secondary References

Ed.Al. (Western suppl.) (1828), 544 and *passim.*
Greenock Trade Directory, passim.
Med.Dir. (1853), 786 and *passim.*

85. Greenock Medical Society (1865–1907*)

History

The early meetings of the Society were held at various locations, including the homes of members, which suggests that it was initially a small organisation. By 1881, the Society rented its own rooms in Kirk Street for meetings and possessed a library. *The Society was the precursor of the Greenock Faculty of Medicine (83), which was established the year of the Society's demise, and although the new Faculty met at a different location, Greenock Infirmary, the day of meeting, the first Wednesday of each month remained the same.

Objects

'... to receive communications on Medicine and Surgery, to converse on medical topics, and generally to promote professional improvement and amicable feelings by any means that from time to time [may] be approved of by the Society'. (*Greenock Trade Directory* (1877), 52)

Membership

No details.

Meetings

Monthly on Mondays, later on Wednesdays, at 8.30 p.m. at the Watt Institution.

Publications

N.I.

Records

N.L.

Secondary References

EMJ 12 (1866–7), 576; 14 (1868–9), 576 ; 16 (1870–1), 672.
Greenock Trade Directory, passim.
Med.Dir., passim.
Year-Book (1884), 158 and *passim.*

86. Greenock Phrenological Society (1833–6>) [L]

History

Two of the Society's twenty-one members in 1836 were medical practitioners. The Society was given impetus by two series of public lectures on phrenology given in 1834/5 and 1835/6 by Professor Robert Hunter (75) and by John Robertson Wood, a general practitioner in Glasgow. The Society possessed a museum of approximately 100 head casts and other items, and also had a small library.

Objects

No details.

Membership

Twenty-one members in 1836.

Meetings

Fortnightly in winter.

Publications

N.I.

Records

N.L.

Secondary References
Watson (1836), 138.

87. Gymnastic Society (1786–1807)

History

This athletic and social club was linked to the Aesculapian Club (7), and like other late eighteenth-century medical clubs was open to both physicians and surgeons. For years the club held annual sporting events including golf, bowls and swimming tournaments for which trophies were presented, but as its members grew less vigorous, the club declined, and at its termination it had become a dining club. The Gymnastic Society's cups, medals and records were passed on to the Aesculapian Club.

Objects

To improve the standards of health and fitness of the profession in the city.

Membership

Consisted of members of the Aesculapian Club and other interested medical practitioners. Thirty members in its early years.

Meetings

Held an annual gymnastic convention at Leith Golf-house, followed by a dinner.

Publications

N.I.

Records

Records and trophies with the records of the Aesculapian Club, in the Library of the Royal College of Physicians, Edinburgh.

Secondary References
Power (1939), 46–7.
EMJ 20/1 (1874), 99–101.

88. Inverness Medical Mission Society (<1866–?) [L]

History

Although established as an auxiliary branch of the Edinburgh Medical Missionary Society (37), the Inverness Society was one of a number of medical missionary societies established throughout Scotland in the middle of the nineteenth century; other societies were set up in Aberdeen (3) and Glasgow (65). Medical Missionary Societies had the dual purpose of providing free medical care for the local population, and also training medical students for overseas medical missionary work. Local medical practitioners were involved as both superintendents of mission dispensaries, and as administrators of the societies. The Inverness Medical Mission Society was addressed at a public meeting in 1866 by the Medical Superintendent of the Edinburgh Society, and by local practitioners, but its ultimate fate is unclear.

Objects

To provide free medical care for local poor, and to train medical students for medical missionary service overseas.

Membership

Open to medical practitioners, and other interested individuals.

Meetings

F.U.

Publications

N.I.

Records

N.L.

Secondary References

Inverness Advertiser, 14 September 1866, 2.

89. Inverness Medical Society (1885–1906)

History

In 1895, the Society worked closely with the Northern Scottish Counties Branch of the BMA to draw attention to the issue of the low level of remuneration involved in club medical practice, which was regarded by the profession as a form of contracted cheap labour. A key role was played in this discussion by the Honorary Secretary of the Inverness Medical Society, and member of the local BMA branch, J. Munro Moir, surgeon at the Northern Infirmary, Inverness, who notified the *BMJ* of the Society's discussions and of its coorrespondence with medical societies in Portsmouth and Cork on the issue of 'the Abuse of Clubs'. As a result of the Society's campaign, all local medical practitioners signed a pledge not to undertake any medical club practice which fell below the Society's agreed minimum level of two shillings and sixpence per head, exclusive of medicines.

Objects

To advance the educational and professional interests of local medical practitioners.

Membership

Open to all qualified practitioners in the locality.

Meetings

Monthly on Mondays at 8 p.m. from October to April.

Publications

N.I.

Records

N.L.

Secondary References

BMJ 2 (1895), 1226, 1440, 1461–2.
Med.Dir. (1898), 1523 and *passim*.
Year-Book (1897), 256 and *passim*.

90. Journal Club (1928–39)

History

The Journal Club was a small medical reading club, which met in the Library of the Royal College of Physicians to discuss articles appearing in a range of contemporary medical journals, and also to discuss predetermined medical subjects in the light of recent medical debate. Occasional meetings were given over to general medical discussion, as in June 1935, when topics raised included the present medical curriculum, and the influx of German practitioners of Jewish origin. The Club also held dinners and other social events. The Journal Club came to an end on the outbreak of the Second World War.

Objects

To discuss matters deemed by the members to be of general medical interest as they arose in contemporary medical journals.

Membership

The Club's average membership was ten, and the number of members was limited to a maximum of twelve.

Meetings

Originally held fortnightly, meetings soon became less frequent, approximately six per year.

Publications

N.I.

Records

Minute book in the Library of the Royal College of Physicians, Edinburgh.

Secondary References

N.I.

91. Kilmarnock Phrenological Society (1826–<36) [L]

History

Although organised phrenological debate had ceased in Kilmarnock sometime before 1836, the science of phrenology still had strong support from the local medical profession. According to Hewett Cottrell Watson's *Statistics of Phrenology* (1836), seven medical practitioners in Kilmarnock had expressed their support for its tenets, including local surgeons, John Crooks, who was a member of the national Phrenological Association, and Alexander Hood, a member of the Glasgow Medical Society who had an 'Essay on Phrenology' read before the Society in 1826. Two medical practitioners were among the original membership of the Kilmarnock Phrenological Society. The dormant Society possessed a small library and a collection of over fifty casts and skulls.

Objects

The progress of phrenological science.

Membership

The Society had between twenty and twenty-four members in its short existence. The admission fee was ten shillings, with a further four shillings to be paid annually.

Meetings

Monthly.

Publications

N.I.

Records

N.L. See MS Essays read before the Glasgow Medical Society vol. 13 February 1826, in the Library of the Royal College of Physicians and Surgeons, Glasgow.

Secondary References

Cooter (1989), 90; 172; 234; 323; 335.
Cottrell Watson (1836), 142.

92. Lanark Medical Society (<1824–7>)

History

There are few details on this Society. John Gibson, a surgeon from Biggar, was the Lanark Society's President; he later became Parochial Medical officer for the district.

Objects

Mutual educational improvement.

Membership

Four office bearers in 1824.

Meetings

F.U.

Publications

N.L.

Records

N.I.

Secondary References

Ed.Al. (Glasgow suppl.) (1824), 494, and *passim*.
Med.Dir,. *passim*.

93. Lothians Medical Association (1868–72)

History

This Association had ambitious professional aims, to enhance the status and increase the level of remuneration of the local profession. The Association was under the Presidency of Robert Christison (82) and included James Young Simpson, (8, 42) and John Hughes Bennett (47) among its membership. The chief method by which these professional goals were to be achieved was through the introduction of a series of binding fee levels for all practitioners in the locality. It was the intention of the Association to gain as many members as possible to ensure any professional policy adopted by the Association would operate across the region. The failure to achieve this end may have led to the premature demise of the Association.

Objects

'... to elevate the whole profession, by elevating the status of the individual members, and at the same time to bind... together [the profession] by more kindly ties of brotherhood and fellowship'. (James Young Simpson, in the chair for a meeting of the Association, 1866)

Membership

Open to all medical practitioners in the Lothians.

Meetings

F.U.

Publications

Report on the Medical Charities of Edinburgh by the Lothians Medical Association (Edinburgh, 1868).
Table of Fees of the Lothian's Medical Association (Edinburgh, 1868).

Records

N.L.

Secondary References

EMJ 12 (1866–7), 952–9; 14 (1868–9), 191–2.

94. Medical and Dental Defence Union of Scotland (1902–extant)

History

The union is a professional defence organisation, which offers insurance and legal protection for qualified medical and dental practitioners. The Union superseded the Edinburgh-based Scottish Medical Defence Association, (114), which was in existence for five years between 1895–9. The formation of the Defence Union came at a time when sections of the medical profession, chiefly in the west of Scotland, were under legal pressure due to their employment of unqualified medical dispensary assistants in their dispensaries, and a number had been recently fined by the courts for allowing unqualified assistants to dispense drugs which was contrary to the Pharmacy Acts. At a meeting of the Glasgow Southern Medical Society (78) to discuss this issue in December 1900, the call was made for 'the formation of a medical defence union' to protect professional interests.

Objects

To protect registered medical and dental practitioners from any liability that may arise in the course of their professional activity.

Membership

It is normal practice for all medical and dental practitioners in Scotland to become members of the Defence Union. Had 6,300 members in 1949.

Meetings

Held in the Union's Buildings in West George Street.

Publications

N.I.

Records

Minute books held at the Medical Defence Union Office, Glasgow.

Secondary References

GMJ 55 (January–June 1901), 133–4.
Med.Dir, passim.

95. Medical and Surgical Institute of Glasgow (1847–1851>)

History

This institution had close links with the medical school at Anderson's University. The Honorary President of the Society was Moses Stephen Buchanan, Professor of Anatomy at Anderson's and Senior Surgeon at Glasgow Royal Infirmary; Andrew Anderson, Professor of the Practice of Medicine, and George Buchanan, Demonstrator in Anatomy, were among the Institute's office-bearers. The Institute's meetings were also held at the University.

Objects

To hear papers on medical subjects, and to hold regular discussions on a variety of medical topics.

Membership

No details as to size. The Institution had ten office-bearers in 1851.

Meetings

Weekly on Mondays during the winter session of the University.

Publications

N.I.

Records

N.L.

Secondary References
Ed.Al. (Western suppl.) (1851), 66.

96. Medical Society of the North (1817–29>)

History

The Society had a library of medical journals for circulation among the members, and also possessed a small collection of morbid specimens. In 1818, the Society published a set of rules for members, which included a schedule of recommended fees for local practitioners, both physicians and surgeons. The schedule was divided into four levels of fees according to social class, which was determined by patient income. In the case of the highest level, the fee level was to be regarded as a minimum to be charged, while among the poorest class, some discretion was to be allowed according to circumstance. For a single consultation the recommended fee charged was to be two shillings and sixpence for the fourth (lowest) class and ten shillings and sixpence for the first (highest) class. The long-serving Secretary of the Society was local Inverness Surgeon, John Inglis Nicol.

Objects

'... promoting Medical Science, and establishing a Professional Library'. (*Inverness Journal*, 9 May 1817)

Membership

Had over thirty members in 1821.

Meetings

Monthly on Tuesdays at 12 o'clock in Inverness in the Society's rooms.

Publications

Rules Adopted by the Medical Society of the North (Inverness, 1818).

Records

N.L.

Secondary References

Ed.Al. (Northern Counties suppl.) (1818), 4 and *passim.*
EMSJ 17 (1821), 317.
Hamilton (1981), 171–2.
Inverness Journal, 9 May 1817, 2 and *passim.*

97. Medico-Chirurgical Society of Dumfries (<1822–4>)

History

The Society was formed by all the medical practitioners in Dumfries out of a feeling that such an institution was an important element in elevating the local profession. Two papers read before the Society in 1822 and 1823 by William Maxwell, a general practitioner based in Langholm, on 'experiments on variolous inoculation' and 'hydrocephalus' were published in the *Edinburgh Medical and Surgical Journal* in 1824.

Objects

'... to cherish the feelings of amity and forbearance, which ought especially to distinguish the profession of so enlightened an art as that of medicine'. (*EMSJ* 18 (1822), 485)

Membership

No details.

Meetings

F.U.

Publications
N.I.
Records
N.L.
Secondary References
EMSJ 18 (1822), 485; 22 (1824), 9, 11.

98. Mentieth Medical Society (1861–?)

History

The Society met in Dunblane, and its origins lay in the grievances of local practitioners over the levels of remuneration they received in the community. To remedy this situation the Society decided to fix a schedule of fees, and also to set aside an hour each day, between 9 and 10 a.m., for free consultations to be given to the local poor. The majority of the Society's members practised in Dunblane and Callander.

Objects

'The mutual advancement of medical knowledge'. (*Stirling Journal,* 19 April 1861)

Membership

Established with twelve founder members.

Meetings

Every second month.

Publications

N.I.

Records

N.L.

Secondary References

Stirling Journal and Advertiser, 19 April 1861, 4.

99. Monklands Medical Society (<1913–15>)

History

In 1913, the Secretary of the Monklands Medical Society, James Andrew, Honorary Surgeon at the Alexander Hospital, Coatbridge, and Medical Officer for the Post Office in Coatbridge, contacted the Scottish Midland and Western Medical Association (115) to ask the latter body to form a committee to consider an ethical dispute which had arisen among the members of the Monklands Society, and to give an opinion on the matter. A small committee was established of the SMWMA's chief office-bearers, but there is no reference to their decision, nor are there any details as to the nature of the dispute. In 1915, the members of the Monklands Society presented James Andrew with a cheque in recognition of his services to the Society, and as Secretary of the Coatbridge Medical and Panel Committees.

Objects

No details available.

Membership

Open to general practitioners in Monklands district.

Meetings

Annual business meeting in April.

Publications

N.I.

Records

N.L. See minute book of the Scottish Midland and Western Medical Association, 26 July 1913.

Secondary References

GMJ 84 (1915), 46–7.

100. North of Scotland Medical Association (1865–92)

History

This Association was originated by the Buchan Medical Society (16), which successfully approached other medical societies in the region, including the Aberdeen Medico-Chirurgical Society (4), the Banff, Moray and Nairn Medical Association (12), and the Garioch and Northern Medical Association (57) in August 1864, to enlist their support for the formation of a regional northern association, with each society retaining its own independent status. The Council of the Association consisted of an annually elected President, plus the Presidents and Secretaries and two nominated delegates from each of the affiliated local medical societies. The Association played a key role in overseeing the professional affairs of local medical practitioners, drawing up a code of medical ethics in 1872 and a uniform table of fees in 1875, and dealing with professional matters remitted to the Association by the local societies, e.g. in September 1869, the Buchan Medical Society submitted the question of the level of fees for medical witnesses to the larger Association.

Objects

'The promotion of friendly intercourse among the Members; the discussions of questions of general or scientific interest to the profession; and the giving expression to the opinion of the Profession in this part of the country on public questions'. (Unnamed local newspaper report of inaugural meeting of NSMA, 5 August 1865, among papers of Garioch and Northern Medical Association)

Membership

All the members of the affiliate societies and interested individual practitioners in the north of Scotland. Annual subscription was two shillings for affiliate members and two shillings and sixpence for individual members. Inaugural meeting attended by sixty seven practitioners from the north of Scotland.

Meetings

Annually in the Hall of the Aberdeen Medico-Chirurgical Society in June or July.

Publications

Report of the Committee on 'Medical Ethics' Appointed by the North of Scotland Medical Association (Inverurie, 1872).

Records

N.L. See printed circulars from the Association among the papers of the Buchan Medical Society, and the Garioch and Northern Medical Association, and also minute books of these societies, *passim*, Manuscripts Collection, Aberdeen University Library.

Secondary References

EMJ 14 (1868–9), 192; 23/1 (1877), 382; 28/2 (1883), 663–4.
Med.Dir., passim.
Year-Book (1884), 158 and *passim*.

101. Northern Counties Medical Association (1863–73)

History

This Association is not to be confused with the North of Scotland Medical Association (100). This shorter-lived Association, which met alternately in Inverness and Elgin, became one of the affiliate members of the NSMA, sending two delegates to the latter's annual conference in Aberdeen. The Association's President in 1872 was John Wilson, Medical Officer at the Northern Infirmary and at Inverness Prison, and Consultant Physician at the District Lunatic Asylum. The President in 1873 was George Duff, Physician at Anderson's Institution, Elgin.

Objects

To represent the social and educational interests of the local profession.

Membership

No precise details. The Association had eleven office-bearers in 1872.

Meetings

Annually in September.

Publications

N.I.

Records

N.L.

Secondary References

Med.Dir., passim.

102. Paisley Medical Society* (1818–extant)

History

The Paisley Medical Society's establishment in 1818 was a reflection of the expansion of the town, as the number of medical practitioners grew to meet the needs of the increasing population. This expansion in professional medical service was shown in the extension of Paisley Dispensary to include a house of recovery in 1805, and a short-lived precursor of the later Society was established in the Dispensary at that time. *Early this century the Society's title was changed to the Paisley Pathological and Clinical Society. The Society is now a social club which holds an annual dinner. The more educational aspect of local medical debate has recently been assumed by the Paisley and District Educational Forum. Female practitioners in the area were admitted to Society membership in 1979.

Objects

'For the mutual communication of professional knowledge and friendly intercourse'. (*Edinburgh Almanac*, 1828)

Membership

Open to all medical practitioners in the district. The Society had forty members in 1824, and the current membership is around 100.

Meetings

The more frequent scientific and professional meetings have been replaced by a well-attended annual dinner, which is addressed by a guest medical speaker.

Publications

N.I.

Records

Current minute book and surviving records are held by the Paisley Pathological and Clinical Society.

Secondary References
Ed.Al. (Western suppl.) (1828), 537, and *passim*.
Dow (1989), 10.

103. Perthshire Medical Association (1879–88*)

History

The Association was formed at a preliminary general meeting of the medical practitioners in the county, when it was decided that such a local representative body was necessary. By the end of 1879, more than half of the practitioners in the district had enrolled in the Association. In 1882, a volume of transactions covering meetings held from 1879–81 was published. In January 1888, the Secretary of the Perthshire body applied to the BMA to be recognised as a branch of the national Association. Twenty five members of the Perthshire Association, who were also members of the BMA signed the petition. *In March 1888, the Association was formally recognised as the Perthshire branch of the BMA.

Objects

'To receive and discuss communications on medicine and surgery and allied subjects, and to promote professional fellowship'. (*Year-Book*, 1884)

Membership

Open to registered medical men in Perth or the adjoining county. Had forty seven members in 1884.

Meetings

Originally held monthly, in Perth Royal Infirmary.

Publications

Transactions of the Perthshire Medical Association (Perth, 1882).

Records

N.L. See Printed Reports of Sub-Committees, BMA Council Minutes, 1889–90, BMA library, London.

Secondary References
EMJ 25/1 (1879), 384.
Lancet 2 (20 September 1879), 445.
Med. Dir. (1881), 1025.
Year-Book (1884), and *passim*.

104. Physico-Chemical Society of Edinburgh (1819–22)

History

There are few details on this Society which was originally listed as the Physico-Chymical Society in the *Edinburgh Almanac*. Benjamin Bell, an Edinburgh surgeon, was President of the Society, and was also a founder member of the Edinburgh Medico-Chirurgical Society (40) in 1821.

Objects

No information available.

Membership

No details as to the size of this Society.

Meetings

F.U.

Publications

N.I.

Records

N.L.

Secondary References

Ed. Al. (1819), 261, and *passim.*

EMJ 19/2 (January–June 1874), 770.

105. Royal Medico-Chirurgical Society of Glasgow (*1814–extant)

History

*The Society was founded in 1866 by the amalgamation of the Glasgow Medical Society (66) with the Medico-Chirurgical Society of Glasgow, established in 1844, from which the new Society derived its name. The newly amalgamated Society adopted 1814 as the date of its foundation, as this was the year in which the Glasgow Medical Society was founded. The amalgamation of the two Glasgow medical societies was a decision made in the interests of each, since the societies had many common members, and their functions were similar, although the Medico-Chirurgical Society of 1844 differed from its older counter-part in that it never had a compulsory element in attendance and the reading of papers. In 1886, the Society was subdivided into sections for the purpose of holding separate meetings on Medicine, Surgery, Pathology and Obstetrics, but this experiment was ended in 1894, the separate sections continuing in name only until the early years of the twentieth century. In 1907, the Glasgow Pathological and Clinical Society (74) was also merged with the Medico-Chirurgical Society. In 1911, the decision was finally taken to admit female practitioners to the Society, after an abortive attempt in 1903 was ruled unconstitutional. During the First World War, Society meetings, including planned centenary celebrations, were suspended; but in 1919, the year in which the delayed centenary celebrations were held, the Society was granted permission to use the prefix 'Royal' in its title.

Objects

'To receive communications on medicine, surgery, and the collateral sciences, and to promote professional improvement'. (*Year-Book*, 1884)

Membership

Candidates for admission to be proposed by two members. Annual subscription was originally five shillings, increased to ten shillings and sixpence in 1924/5, later reduced to seven shillings in 1934/5. Twenty-six ordinary members in 1844, rose to over 200 in 1884, and to 398 in 1902, but fell to 316 in 1932/3, and was down to 240 in 1934/5.

Meetings

Held at 8 p.m. on the first Friday of the month from September to May in the Hall of the Faculty of Physicians and Surgeons, Glasgow.

Publications

Transactions of the Medico-Chirurgical Society of Glasgow at first published biannually from 1897 to 1912, thereafter published annually.

Records

Minute books and other records held in the Library of the Royal College of Physicians and Surgeons, Glasgow.

Secondary References

Christie (1888), 181–3.

Dow (1989).
Walker Downie (1907).
Duncan (1896), 192–3.
Power (1939), 63–77.
Thomson, 'Royal Medico-Chirurgical Society of Glasgow' (1976), 168–74.
See also *EMJ, GMJ, Med.Dir.*, and *Year-Book, passim.*

106. Royal Odonto-Chirurgical Society of Scotland (1868–extant)

History

A scientific and professional organisation open to dental surgeons, the Society held a series of preliminary meetings in 1867, although 1868 is the date given for its formal establishment in Edinburgh. The Scottish Branch of the British Dental Association, set up in 1882, represents the political interests of dental practitioners. Before the 1878 Dentists Act, and indeed beyond, many of the early members of the Society were medical practitioners, e.g. in 1872, the President of the Society was Peter Orphoot who was listed in the *Medical Directory* for that year as a 'Surgeon-Dentist'. For many years the Society met in Chambers Street, where it had its own library and reading room. The early practice of the Society was to hear a paper, and have members ask questions of it at the succeeding meeting, when all members would have a printed copy of the paper before them.

Objects

'To promote and diffuse knowledge in matters connected with dental surgery'. (*Year-Book*, 1884)

Membership

Open to qualified dental surgeons, through a ballot. Founded with thirteen members, the Society had seventy members in 1884. Original fee was one guinea for resident members, this figure was reduced to ten shillings for all members in 1896.

Meetings

Monthly from November to March.

Publications

N.L.

Records

Minute books in the Library of the Royal College of Surgeons, Edinburgh.

Secondary References

BMJ 1 (1912), 641 and *passim.*
Menzies Campbell (1958), 105–6, 144–58, 242, 248.
EMJ 15 (1869–70), 142–43, and *passim.*
Ed.Al. (1872), 878 and *passim.*
Year-Book (1884), 156 and *passim.*

107. Royal Society of Edinburgh (1783–extant) [L]

History

The Royal Society of Edinburgh was the direct successor of the Edinburgh Philosophical Society (45), although it was from its foundation, a broader based institution, modelled on continental academies of science and culture, and in possession of a Royal Charter. Originally divided into two groups, the Literary and the Physical, the Royal Society aimed to attract the cream of Scottish scientific and literary talent, and in the early days of the Society, many of its leading members were medical men. In October 1783, for example, those elected Fellows of the Society included: Joseph Black, Professor of Chemistry at Edinburgh University; William Cullen, Professor of the Practice of Physic; Alexander Monro *secundu*s, Professor of Anatomy and Surgery; and Andrew Duncan senior (7, 35, 40). While in 1797 and 1798 respectively, Andrew Duncan junior, Professor of Materia Medica and Pharmacy, and Alexander Monro *tertius*, who had succeeded his father as Professor of Anatomy, were elected to the Fellowship. After 1798, the Literary section was dropped, and the Society came to be predominantly a scientific society. It is now more comprehensive, though this is very recent.

Objects

To cultivate 'every branch of science, erudition, and taste'. (*Transactions of the Royal Society of Edinburgh* 1 (1788), 7)

Membership

The Society has always had a substantial membership. There were 418 Ordinary Fellows in 1884, and this number had risen to 720 in 1937. In 1884, the admission fee was two guineas, and the annual subscription fee was three guineas.

Meetings

On the first and third Monday of each month between November and July. Statutory meeting on the fourth Monday in October.

Publications

Transactions of the Royal Society of Edinburgh and *Proceedings of the Royal Society of Edinburgh*.

Records

Held by the Royal Society of Edinburgh.

Secondary References

History of Science and Medicine Unit, (Edinburgh) *Scotland's Cultural Heritage, Vol. 1* (1981).
History of Science and Medicine Unit, (Edinburgh) *Scotland's Cultural Heritage Vol. 3* (1982).
McElroy (1952), 334–40.
McElroy (1969), 77–80.
Shapin (1971), *passim*.
Shapin, 'Property, patronage, and the politics of science: the founding of the Royal Society of Edinburgh' (1974), 1–41.
See *Ed.Al.* and *Year-Book, passim*.

108. Sanitary Association of Scotland* (1875–extant) [L]

History

The Society was formed as a result of a preliminary meeting of sanitary inspectors in 1874 convened by John Welsh, Superintendent of Police and Sanitary Inspector for Perth. The first President of the Society was Kenneth McLeod, Sanitary Inspector for Glasgow. For the first three years the Society was open only to sanitary inspectors, but after 1878 its membership was broadened, and as the Society's functions evolved, examinations for those interested in becoming Sanitary Inspectors were introduced. The Society also aimed at increasing awareness on matters of public health through popular lectures, and it monitored Government and local legislation on sanitation. Papers relating to sanitary conditions in Scotland were read at the Society's annual congresses. In 1895, for example, at the annual congress in Greenock, Matthew Hay, Medical Officer of Health in Aberdeen, and Physician at the City Hospital, Aberdeen, discussed the rates of mortality in Scotland in relation to sanitary progress, while in 1901, Archibald Kerr

Chalmers, Medical Officer of Health for the City of Glasgow, discussed the control of dairies and the supply of milk. *The Society was given a 'Royal' prefix in 1925, and had also previously been known as the Incorporated Sanitary Association of Scotland. In 1983, the Royal Sanitary Association of Scotland was amalgamated with the Scottish Institute of Environmental Health to form the Royal Environmental Health Institute of Scotland.

Objects

'... the mutual consideration of subjects connected with sanitary matters; the diffusion of information which will lead to increased knowledge of the laws of health, and sanitary science generally; the establishing of a proper system of co-operation and communication between sanitary inspectors throughout Scotland...'. (Christie (1888), 191)

Membership

Open to sanitary inspectors, interested medical practitioners, and lay persons. The original membership fee was two shillings and sixpence. The Society had 405 members in 1913, 320 in 1964.

Meetings

Originally held when necessary, with an annual meeting in the autumn. The annual meeting was expanded to a three-day annual Congress. Meetings held around Scotland.

Publications

Sanitary Journal published after 1876.
Transactions of the Sanitary Association of Scotland.

Records

N.L.

Secondary References

Christie (1888), 190–2.
Lancet 2 (1901), 620, 762; 2 (1913), 894–5 and *passim*.
Year-Book (1891), 207 and *passim*.

109. Scottish Association for Mental Health (1921–extant) [L]

History

The Edinburgh-based Association was set up to promote interest in mental health matters, and offers an advisory service to those with mental health problems. It also possesses a reference library of related medical works.

Objects

'To foster a wider understanding throughout the country of the importance of mental health in every day life and to spread the knowledge of the ways by which mental health may be achieved and maintained and mental ill health or disability prevented'. (*Year-Book*, 1964)

Membership

Open to medical practitioners and interested lay persons.

Meetings

F.U.

Publications

Various reports, periodical and pamphlets.

Records

N.L.

Secondary References
Year-Book (1964), 97.

110. Scottish Branch, British Homoeopathic Society* (<1921–extant)

History

Although not strictly a Scottish medical society, this local branch of a national British association is entered here in an attempt to provide as comprehensive a picture as possible of the complexion of Scottish medical society activity in the period, including the area of complementary medicine. *The Society became known as the Scottish Branch of the British Homoeopathic Society and Faculty of Homoeopathy in 1938.

Objects

To hear papers and case studies, and to discuss matters of prevailing medical interest.

Membership

Open to homoeopathic medical practitioners in Scotland.

Meetings

F.U.

Publications

N.I.

Records

Held in the Faculty of Homoeopathy, Glasgow Homoeopathic Library.

Secondary References

N.I.

111. Scottish Eastern Association of Medical Women* (1899–extant)

History

*The Association was known as the Edinburgh Medical Women's Club until 1906, and until 1918, as the Scottish Association of Medical Women. Under its present title it became part of the national Medical Women's Federation. The original club was set up by the small group of female medical graduates of the Edinburgh Extra-Mural Medical School at the end of the nineteenth century. Among them were Jessie MacGregor, Registrar and Assistant to the Extra Physician, Royal Hospital for Sick Children, Edinburgh, and Elsie Inglis, Gynaecologist at St. Anne's Dispensary, Edinburgh, who set up practice together after their graduation. Elsie Inglis later became Physician to the Scottish Hospital Unit (which served in France and Serbia during the First World War), and served as President of the Scottish Association of Medical Women from 1913 until her death in 1918. In 1899, the Edinburgh Medical Women's Club established a small nursing home for female patients, and in 1910 the home was united with the Bruntsfield Women's Hospital (set up in 1878 by Sophia Jex-Blake), which continued until 1924 when it was superseded by the Elsie Inglis Memorial Maternity Hospital. In 1916, the hospital offered facilities for study for female medical students on their admission to the medical faculty of Edinburgh University. The Edinburgh Medical Women's Club is not to be confused with the student Edinburgh Women's Medical Society (entry 13 in student society list) set up in 1913. From 1918 until 1932, when it was disbanded, the Scottish regional medical federations met under the name of the Scottish Union of Medical Women (125), to discuss affairs affecting the Scottish female medical profession. The Eastern Scottish Association holds an annual clinical meeting with the Scottish Western Association (58).

Objects

To promote and protect the professional interests of female medical practitioners.

Membership

Twelve known members at the turn of the century.

Meetings

Monthly during the Edinburgh University term at the Pfeizer Institute Post-graduate Medical Centre, Hill Square, Edinburgh.

Publications

N.I.

Records

Incomplete records held by the Scottish Eastern Association of Medical Women. See also Medical Women's Federation papers (SA/MWF c. 3; c.89–90, and MWF Council Minutes May 25 1918) in Contemporary Archives, Wellcome Institute Library, London.

Secondary References

Med.Dir,. passim.
Year-Book (1913), 371 and *passim.*

112. Scottish Medical Defence Association Limited* (1895–9)

History

*The Association should not be confused with the Medical and Dental Defence Union of Scotland (94), which was set up in 1902. In 1898, Norman Walker, Assistant Physician in Dermatology at Edinburgh Royal Infirmary, later elected as the Scottish directly-elected member of the General Medical Council in 1901, was President of this Edinburgh-based professional defence Association.

Objects

To protect registered medical practitioners from legal liability in professional matters.

Membership

Open to all qualified medical practitioners in Scotland.

Meetings

Held as required. The Annual meeting was in April.

Publications

N.I.

Records

N.L.

Secondary References

Med.Dir. (1898), 1522.
Year-Book (1898), 269.

113. Scottish Medico-Psychological Association (<1902–?)

History

There is little information extant on this Association, other than a reference to it in the Council Minutes of the Edinburgh Medico-Chirurgical Association in 1902. This stated that all members of the Scottish Medico-Psychological Association were to be invited to a special meeting of the Medico-Chirurgical Society to be held in Edinburgh Royal Infirmary to discuss the treatment of incipient forms of insanity.

Objects
No details.
Membership
Open to medical practitioners with an interest in psychology.
Meetings
F.U.
Publications
N.I.
Records
N.L. See Edinburgh Medico-Chirurgical Society Council minute book, 5 February 1902 (MAC GD 3/2/3) in Special Collections, Edinburgh University Library.
Secondary References
N.I.

114. Scottish Microscopical Society (1889–1921) [L]
History
The Scottish Microscopical Society was set up in Edinburgh by a group of medical practitioners and members of the medical faculty of Edinburgh University. The Society's first President was Sir William Turner, Professor of Anatomy at Edinburgh University, and member of the General Medical Council. After many years of flourishing existence, when regular annual volumes of proceedings were produced, the Society was eventually brought to a close through lack of interest in 1921.
Objects
The discussion of problems connected with the use of microscopy in medicine and science.
Membership
Open to medical practitioners and other interested individuals. Formed with 102 members.
Meetings
Monthly on Fridays at 8 p.m. from November to March.
Publications
Transactions of the Scottish Microscopical Society, later became *Proceedings of the Scottish Microscopical Society*
Records
Minute books in Special Collections, Edinburgh University Library.
Secondary References
BMJ 1 (1889), 1477.
Finlayson (1956–8), 19.
Nuttall, 'Early Scottish Microscopes' (1981), 199–200.
Year-Book (1891), 112–13 and *passim*.

115. Scottish Midland and Western Medical Association (1872–extant)
History
The Association for many years had a strong professional and medico-political interest, and indeed, its local branches sought to coordinate professional activity in the counties of

Lanark, Stirling, Clackmannan, Dunbarton, Renfrew, Ayr and Linlithgow. In 1874 the Association, in connection with the Clackmannan and Kinross-shire Medical Association (20), campaigned for the creation of a Scottish Medical Association to protect the whole Scottish profession's interests, but this proposal did not receive sufficient support from other Scottish societies to be put into practice. The Association was concerned with legislation which affected the profession, and also sought to enhance practitioners' fees for public appointments. Medical papers were read before the Association, but these remained secondary to medico-political and professional activities. The Association often sent deputations to London to petition parliament on medical matters, and to speak to political figures involved in the particular legislation, e.g. in 1887, two members were sent to interview the local MP for North-East Lanarkshire, Donald Crawford, with reference to his proposed Truck Law Amendment Act, which was viewed as a threat to the incomes of medical practitioners employed in mining districts. Again, in 1911 the Association decided to send a deputation to interview Lloyd George, the Chancellor of the Exchequer, on various aspects of the National Insurance Bill, particularly how it would affect practitioners involved in works practices, although this approach to the Chancellor was subsequently declined. In 1920, the Association's constitution was amended and meetings became annual, and exclusively social, as they continue to be to the present day.

Objects

'The preservation of the rights and advancement of the interests of the medical profession; the promotion of good fellowship and social intercourse amongst the members; the cultivation of medical, surgical, and sanitary science'. (*Year-Book*, 1884)

Membership

Open to registered male practitioners in the catchment area of the Association. Membership has always averaged around fifty. Original subscription was five shillings a year.

Meetings

Initially council meetings were held quarterly, with an AGM and dinner and special general meetings, all of which were held in Glasgow. The Association now meets annually. Frequency of the short-lived local branch meetings is unknown.

Publications

N.I.

Records

Minute book held by the Honorary Secretary of the Scottish Midland and Western Medical Association.

Secondary References

EMJ 20/1 (1874), 570–571 and *passim*.
See also *Med.Dir.* and *Year-Book*, *passim*.

116. Scottish Opthalmological Club (1911–extant)

History

The Club was originally open only to those holding hospital Opthalmological appointments; but, within a year this restriction was lifted, and all interested practitioners became eligible for membership. The first female practitioners were admitted as members in 1919. The Club had and maintains, a strong social element with papers delivered in an informal manner, and meetings succeeded by a dinner. Until 1925, the only office-bearer of the Club was its Secretary, but since that date a President has been elected annually.

Objects

'To hold friendly meetings occasionally for the exhibition of clinical cases and similar work, for informal interchange of opinions, and for the cultivation of personal acquaintance among those practising our branch of the profession'. (Circular inviting individuals to the Club's first meeting, quoted in Wright Thomson, (1978?))

Membership

Twenty-one members attended the Club's inaugural meeting, this rose to forty two members by 1912, and seventy two in 1929. Original subscription was two shillings and sixpence, raised to ten shillings in 1955, and £1 in 1973.

Meetings

Held around the country, usually twice a year.

Publications

Wright Thomson, *History of the Scottish Opthalmological Club* (1979).

Records

Minute books held by the Scottish Opthalmological Club.

Secondary References

Wright Thomson (1963), 73, 81.

117. Scottish Otological and Laryngological Society (1910–24>)

History

Membership of the Society was restricted to those holding a hospital,. dispensary, or university appointment in this branch of medicine. The first meeting of the Society was held in November 1910 at the Royal Infirmary, Edinburgh, under the chairmanship of Arthur Logan Turner, Consultant Surgeon at the Eye, Ear, and Throat Infirmary, Edinburgh, and Lecturer in Diseases of the Ear and Throat at Edinburgh University. At this inaugural meeting numerous patients were shown, cases were reported and notes read, and a general discussion followed. The meeting was concluded by dinner. In 1924, the Otological and Laryngological Society held a conjoint meeting with the Scottish Opthalmological Club (116) in Edinburgh, on optic neuritis and its connection with diseases of nasal sinuses.

Objects

No details.

Membership

The Society was founded with twenty four members.

Meetings

Held twice a year, one in Edinburgh, the other in Glasgow.

Publications

N.I.

Records

N.L.

Secondary References

EMJ 1 (1911), 3–4.
GMJ 74 (July–December 1910), 445 and passim.
Lancet 2 (1910), 1700–1.
Wright Thomson (1979), 15.

118. Scottish Paediatric Society* (1922–1972>)

History

*The Society was known as the Edinburgh and Glasgow Paediatric Club from 1922–46. The Club was instigated by the senior physicians at the two children's hospitals, John Thomson and J. Stuart Fowler in Edinburgh, and Leonard Findlay in Glasgow. The inaugural meeting of the Club was held at the Royal Sick Children's Hospital in Glasgow. The Club remained an informal gathering, with no office bearers other than a Secretary, and no regular subscriptions. Initially, cases were shown and short papers read, with a break for tea, but after 1927, meetings of the Club were convened after a dinner for members and invited guests. After the Society's name change in 1946, membership was extended to paediatricians around the country, and office-bearers were elected for the first time.

Objects

'... the intercourse of men interested in the medical diseases of children'. (From Society's rules, reproduced in Coleman (1972))

Membership

Ten founder members in 1922, twenty three members in 1945, sixty in 1962, eighty seven in 1972.

Meetings

Twice a year, initially in Edinburgh and Glasgow, after 1946 around the country.

Publications

Coleman, *The Scottish Paediatric Society, 1922–1972* (1972).

Records

N.L.

Secondary References

N.I.

119. Scottish Poor Law Medical Officers Association (1895–1946)

History

It is surprising that there was no specific association to protect the interests of Scottish Poor Law Medical Officers before 1895, since this section of the medical profession had few rights, no fixity of tenure, and were subject to the control of local parochial boards, and bearing in mind that there was an Association for English Poor Law Medical Officers since the 1870s. Before 1895, parochial medical officers had secured some representation of their interests through the work of the BMA in this area of medical employment, and also through local medical society support, but often this was on an individual basis, and the creation of a representative Scottish organisation was overdue. The professional activities of the Scottish Poor Law Medical Officers Association may be illustrated by the fact that in 1901, the annual report of the committee of the Association appealed to all members of the Association to write to their MP's in support of the Bill to amend the Local Government (Scotland) Act which included a clause giving Medical Officers fixity of tenure. The Association provided descriptions of the duties of advertised Poor Law appointments for interested applicants, using information supplied by outgoing medical officers, and also gave advice to parochial medical officers who were experiencing difficulties in their posts. The first Honorary President of the Association was William Bruce of Dingwall, then the directly-elected Scottish representative on the General Medical Council.

Objects

To promote the professional interests of parochial medical officers, including campaigning for fixity of tenure for appointments.

Membership

Open to all practitioners with an interest in Poor Law work, more especially past and present holders of parochial medical appointments.

Meetings

Annually in January in Glasgow.

Publications

N.I.

Records

N.L.

Secondary References

BMJ 1 (1901), 177.
GMJ 77 (1912), 134.
Lancet 1 (1896), 429, 438; 1 (1901), 204, 272 and *passim*.
Little (1932), 105.
See also *Med.Dir.* and *Year-Book, passim.*

120. Scottish Radiological Society (1936–extant)

History

The Society is divided into two sections: radiodiagnosis, and radiotherapy and oncology. Membership of the Society is open to all registered medical practitioners ordinarily engaged in the practice of these branches of Radiology and allied sciences, and to those formerly employed in these areas. The first President of the Society was John Struthers Fulton, Assistant Radiologist at Edinburgh Royal Infirmary. As with many medical societies, the activities of the Radiological Society were curtailed during the Second World War, with office-bearers remaining in post for the duration. President of the Society at this time was John Burnett King, Honorary Radiologist at Leith Hospital and Deaconess Hospital, and Consultant Radiologist for Edinburgh Corporation Hospitals.

Objects

'... to encourage the study and promote the practice of all branches of [Radiology]... and to promote measures affecting any matters connected with them as may be deemed expedient by the Society'. (Constitution of the Scottish Radiological Society, 1986)

Membership

Current membership is approximately 330, no details of previous membership. Annual subscription was originally £2, is now £5 for consultants and £2 for junior staff.

Meetings

Three times per year. The annual meeting is held in November alternately in Edinburgh and Glasgow. The Spring and Summer meetings are held at other parts of the country.

Publications

Constitution of the Scottish Radiological Society (Edinburgh, 1986).

Records

Minute books held by the Archivist, Scottish Radiological Society.

Secondary References

SMJ, passim.

121. Scottish Society of Anaesthetists (1914–extant)

History

The founder members of the Society, although all practising anaesthetists, were also general practitioners, at a time when medical speciality was not necessarily a full-time occupation, and in fact, the first resident anaesthetist was not appointed in Scotland until 1937. The Society did not meet from April 1914 until 1919 due to the prevailing war-time conditions, having had only one formal meeting before war was declared. In 1926, the Society held a joint meeting with the Associated Anaesthetists of the United States and Canada, attended by seven North American anaesthetists. In 1931, Winifred Wood became the first female President of the Society, which from its origin had admitted female practitioners. In 1939, the Society again ceased to meet due to the wartime situation, and was not reconstituted until 1950.

Objects

'To further the study of the science and practice of anaesthetics, and the proper teaching thereof.' (*GMJ*, 1914)

Membership

Limited to those practising the speciality of anaesthetics, but other interested members of the profession can be admitted as guests. Founded with fourteen members.

Meetings

Twice yearly, in April and October, in rotation in Edinburgh, Glasgow, Dundee and Aberdeen.

Publications

Newsletter of the Scottish Society of Anaesthetists, superseded by the *Annals of the Scottish Society of Anaesthetists* (1960–).

Records

Presently held by the current Honorary Secretary in the Western Infirmary, Glasgow.

Secondary References

GMJ (1914), 289.

122. Scottish Society for Experimental Medicine (1938–extant)

History

The Society was initially very exclusive, open only to those holding academic appointments in Scotland's four medical schools, although it is now open to other medical practitioners, including general practitioners. The Society's inaugural meeting in the Clinical Laboratory of Edinburgh Royal Infirmary was attended by twenty-six members. In the first years of the Society's existence, the spread of membership was in relation to the numeric strength of the four medical schools. Additional membership was extended only to invited guests who had presented a paper before the Society, and the presentation of a paper before the Society remains a prerequisite for membership. Also in the early days of the Society, any member who failed to attend meetings on three consecutive occasions was considered to have withdrawn from the Society. Since 1956, regular reports of the Society's proceedings have appeared in the *Scottish Medical Journal* which is co-funded by the Society, £5 of the Society's membership fee going to meet the costs of the journal's publication.

Objects

To provide a scientific forum for discussions and presentations on experimental medicine.

Membership

Initially limited to forty members, the Society had 115 members in 1955. Membership fee was originally ten shillings and stood at £10 in 1988.

Meetings

Held once per academic term, in rotation at the four Scottish medical schools, Edinburgh, Glasgow, Aberdeen and St. Andrews.

Publications

Scottish Society for Experimental Medicine Golden Jubilee Meeting (pamphlet) (Glasgow, 1988).

Records

Minute books held by the current Honorary Secretary of the Scottish Society for Experimental Medicine.

Secondary References

SMJ, passim.

123. Scottish Curative Mesmeric Association (1853–62>) [L]

History

The first President of the Association was William Gregory, Professor of Chemistry at Edinburgh University from 1844–56. One of the directors of the Curative Mesmeric Association was David Brodie, a former Physician-Superintendent of the Scottish Institute for the Education of Imbeciles, and founder of a private home for young imbeciles. Brodie, like Gregory, was also a member of the Edinburgh Phrenological Society (46). Other members included Sir Walter Calverly Trevelyan, Fellow of the Royal Society of Edinburgh (107). In 1861, the Glasgow Curative Mesmeric Assocation (60) was affiliated to the Scottish Association. President of the Scottish Curative Mesmeric Association in 1862 was John Elliotson, an Edinburgh graduate and former Professor of Practical and Clinical Medicine at University College, London, who was also a member of the Edinburgh Phrenological Society.

Objects

To promote interest in the medical applications of mesmerism, or 'medical hypnotism'.

Membership

No details.

Meetings

F.U.

Publications

N.I.

Records

N.L.

Secondary References

Cooter (1989), 38, 154, 327–8.
First Annual Report of the Glasgow Curative Mesmeric Association (1862), 1–2.

124. Scottish Thoracic Society* (1921–extant)

History

*The Society was known as the Tuberculosis Society of Scotland until 1963. The inaugural meeting of the Society was held at the Royal College of Physicians in Edinburgh, where Sir Robert Philip, Senior Physician at Edinburgh Royal Infirmary, and at the Royal Victoria Consumption Hospital, was elected first President, a position he held until 1933. With the decline in the prevalence of tuberculosis in Scotland, the Society's interests were expanded to cover all aspects of respiratory medicine, including related disciplines such as cardiothoracic surgery, anaesthesia, and pathology.

Objects

'... to bring together for purposes of co-operation and discussion members of the Profession resident in Scotland who are interested in Tuberculosis from the medical, surgical, pathological, statistical or administrative point of view, and to stimulate observation and research along the numerous lines which have their common centre in Tuberculosis'. (Minutes of the Tuberculosis Society of Scotland, 1921)

Membership

Open to all persons qualified in Medicine, resident in Scotland. The Society's present membership is around 200. The original membership fee was ten shillings and sixpence.

Meetings

Originally between October and July, at not less than two-month intervals. The Society currently meets twice a year.

Publications

N.L.

Records

Minute books in the Royal College of Physicians, Edinburgh.

Secondary References

See *Med.Dir.* and *Year-Book, passim.*

125. Scottish Union of Medical Women (1919–32)

History

This body was created by members of the Scottish Eastern (111) and Western (58) and branches of the Medical Women's Federation, for the purpose of representing the professional and educational interests of female medical practitioners in Scotland. The Union of Medical Women met independently of the MWF until 1932 when it was replaced by a Scottish standing committee of the national Federation. The reason given for the Union's demise was the drain on the separate Association's finances caused by convening the Scottish meetings, in particular with the creation of the Aberdeen and North of Scotland Association of Medical Women in 1926 (1), which had increased the cost of travelling to meetings. This situation led to a successful proposal to replace the Union with a Scottish standing committee of six delegates from the three Scottish Associations, i.e. the Scottish Council members of the MWF, to meet at the time of the general Council meetings of the MWF in London.

Objects

To represent the interests of medical women in Scotland.

Membership

Open to members of the Scottish Eastern and Western branches of the MWF. Also open to members of the Aberdeen and East of Scotland branch of the MWF after its creation in 1926.

Meetings

Twice yearly.

Publications

N.I.

Records

N.L. See Medical Women's Federation records, Contemporary Archives, Wellcome Institute Library, London, SA/MWF Council Minutes, 25 May 1918; 4 November 1932.

Secondary References

Med.Dir. (1922), 1531 and *passim.*

Year-Book (1920), 341 and *passim.*

126. Society of Licentiates in Dental Surgery (1880–?)

History

This Society was apparently formed due to dissatisfaction among West of Scotland dental surgeons at the unrepresentative nature of the Odonto-Chirurgical Society of Scotland (106), which it was alleged by the Society's first President, James R. Brownlie, a member of the Odonto-Chirurgical Society since 1869, had settled for protecting the interests of its resident Edinburgh members.

Objects

To represent the professional interests of Scottish Licentiates in Dental Surgery.

Membership

No figures or details available.

Meetings

F.U.

Publications

N.L.

Records

N.L.

Secondary References

Menzies Campbell (1959), 155.

127. Society of Medical Officers of Health for Scotland (1891–1908)

History

Archibald Campbell Munro, County Medical Officer of Health for Renfrewshire, and Honorary Secretary of the Society from 1891–7, was responsible for convening the first meeting of Scottish Medical Officers of Health in April 1891, and the Society met formally for the first time at the Royal College of Surgeons in Edinburgh in July. In 1896, the Society was affiliated to the Incorporated Society of Medical Officers of Health, but continued to meet separately as an independent body for some years, with Society office-bearers holding the same position at both Society and Branch level. In 1908, the Society formally became a branch of the British Society of Medical Officers of Health, which continued to meet until 1976.

Objects

To coordinate the effort of those responsible for protecting the public health in Scotland.

Membership

Thirteen Scottish Medical Officers attended the first meeting, with a further nine expressing written support for the Society.

Meetings

On the last Friday in March, June and September; in Glasgow, Perth, and Edinburgh alternately.

Publications

N.I.

Records

N.L.

Secondary References

Med.Dir., passim.
Year-Book (1894), 221 and *passim.*
Tait, 'Notes on the Scottish Branch of the Society of Medical Officers of Health' (1976), 265–70.

128. Statistical Society of Glasgow (1836–46?) [L]

History

Although this Society was a general statistical society, it had a strong medical presence at a period when the use of statistics in investigations into disease was increasingly employed as a method of expanding medical knowledge and of assessing public health patterns. In 1838, four of the Society's eight office bearers were medical practitioners, including Robert Cowan, Physician at Glasgow Fever Hospital, and Robert Perry, Physician at Glasgow Royal Infirmary, who were both council members.

Objects

'To collect, arrange, and publish, facts illustrative of the condition and prosperity of the nation, with a view to the improvement of mankind'. (*Journal of the Statistical Society of London*, 1838)

Membership

No figures available.

Meetings

F.U.

Publications

N.I.

Records

N.L.

Secondary References

Cullen (1975), 119–20, 121.
Ed.Al. (Western suppl.) (1838), 67, and *passim.*
Eyler (1979), 13, 29–31.
Journal of the Statistical Society of London 1 (June 1838), 115.

129. Stirling Medical Association (1836–50>)

History

The Association met in the Stirling Dispensary, and for the first few years of its existence its functions remained medico-scientific and educational, hearing papers from local practitioners, and building up its medical library. In June 1840, however, the Association placed an advertisement in the *Stirling Journal and Advertiser* announcing a special meeting of all practitioners in the area to draw up a petition to Parliament on the matter of medical reform. The issue of the reform of medical education in Britain, in an attempt to exclude unqualified practitioners, and enhance the status of those fully qualified through the creation of a medical register, was at this time a key one in medical professional debate, and many societies around the country were promoting the cause of medical reform, including the Eastern (30) and Western (134) Medical Associations of Scotland. The increasing involvement of medical societies in medico-political affairs is exemplified by the Stirling Medical Association's decision to call a public meeting and draw up a petition to Parliament on the issue. The President of the Association in 1850 was William Ross, a former Royal Navy Surgeon.

Objects

To hear communications on medical subjects and to provide a medical library.

Membership

Open to any medical practitioner residing in Stirlingshire, Clackmannanshire, and west Perthshire. Subscription fee was one guinea. Thirty founder members.

Meetings

On the first Friday of each month.

Publications

N.I.

Records

N.L.

Secondary References

EMSJ 54 (1840), 535–6.
Stirling Journal and Advertiser, 8 January 1836 and *passim*.

130. Stirling Medical Society (1889–1909>)

History

The Society sought to create the atmosphere of a small reading club for its members, and to hold informal meetings to discuss professional matters in a social manner. It also discussed matters of local medical interest. In 1909, the Society drew up a report on the invitation of the local Public Health Committee on the more effective management of pulmonary phthisis in the district, the result of which was to rule out the immediate construction of a consumption hospital on the grounds of cost. Three months later, John Drew, a former Surgeon in HM Prison Stirling, the Society's Secretary and Treasurer, revived the issue in the local press by suggesting that an empty building in Friar Street, Stirling would provide a satisfactory site for the location of such a hospital. It is unclear whether this proposal met with other than editorial support, and there is no indication as to the subsequent fate of the Society itself.

Objects

'... for the promotion of friendly feeling and social intercourse among the members, and the discussion of scientific and medical subjects'. (*Stirling Journal*, August 1888)

Membership

Sixteen founder members.

Meetings

F.U.

Publications

N.I.

Records

N.L.

Secondary References
Cook and Wylie's *Stirling Directory* (1901), 210 and *passim.*
Harvey's *Stirling Directory and Almanack* (1889), 85.
Stirling Journal and Advertiser, 12 July 1888, 4.

131. Town and Country Club (1893–6>)

History

The Club was established to cater for the social interests of medical practitioners in Glasgow and its surrounding districts. Unlike the older Western Medical Club (135), which pursued similar objects, the Town and Country Club did not have a fixed limit on membership, and it is this fact which led to its creation.

Objects

To provide opportunities for regular and friendly intercourse between members of the profession in Glasgow and the West of Scotland.

Membership

No details.

Meetings

F.U.

Publications

N.I.

Records

N.L.

Secondary References
Duncan (1896), 198.

132. Wernerian Natural History Society (1808–58) [L]

History

This prestigious natural history society named after geologist, Adam Gottlob Werner, had many medical members including Alexander Monro *tertius*, Professor of Anatomy at Edinburgh University, Robert Knox, extra-mural lecturer in Anatomy, and James Syme, lecturer in Anatomy at the time of his admission, later Professor of Clinical Surgery at Edinburgh University. Having obtained a 'Seal of Cause' incorporating the Society from Edinburgh Town Council shortly after its foundation in 1808, the Wernerian soon established a worldwide reputation in natural science, and in 1811 had 110 overseas corresponding members. In the 1830s, the Society offered a series of prizes of 10 and 20 sovereigns for the best essays on natural scientific subjects which were also published in the Society's transactions. The Wernerian Society's international reputation declined and the number of its foreign corresponding members was greatly reduced after it ceased the publication of its transactions in 1839. Meetings of the Society became less frequent in the late 1840s and it did not meet after November 1850. In 1858, the Society was formally disbanded, with its remaining members, museum and book collection divided between the Edinburgh Botanical Society (15) and the Edinburgh Royal Physical Society (51).

Objects

The advancement of general natural history, but more especially the natural history of Scotland.

Membership

The Society had forty-four Resident members in 1811, and seventy in 1853. Membership fee was one guinea.

Meetings

Originally fortnightly on Saturdays, later meetings were held monthly.

Publications

Memoirs of the Wernerian Natural History Society (8 vols, Edinburgh/London 1811–39).

Records

Minute books in Special Collections, Edinburgh University Library.

Secondary References

Finlayson (1956–8), 19.
Hume (1853), 175.
Med.Dir. (1853), 789.
Proceedings of the Royal Physical Society (Vol. 2, 1863), 11–12.

133. Western Infirmary Residents' Club (1895–1935>)

History

The Club was formally convened in February 1895 at an annual dinner for past and present residents of Glasgow Western Infirmary, after meeting on an informal basis since 1886. The Club was open to all men who were or had been Resident Assistants or Superintendents in the Infirmary. There were no female residents at the Western in the period from its opening in 1874 to 1935 when a list of residents was published by the Club.

Objects

'...to promote friendly intercourse amongst its members.'

Membership

Over seventy members attended the 1911 and 1922 dinners. The annual subscription was 2 shillings and 6 pence or one guinea for life membership.

Meetings

Annual business meeting and dinner in February.

Publications

Western Infirmary Residents' Club List of Members 1874–1935 (Glasgow, 1935).

Records

N.L.

Secondary References

BMJ 1 (1911), 395.
GMJ 79 (1913), 201; 98 (1922), 173–4 and *passim*.

134. Western Medical Association* (1839–40>)

History

The Western Medical Association sent delegates to the London congresses on medical reform held at Exeter Hall in 1840/1. The whole movement for the reform of medical education was given impetus by the introduction of three, albeit unsuccessful, private member's bills on medical reform before parliament in 1840–1, and it is no coincidence that the Eastern Medical Association of Scotland (30) was also active in medical politics at this period. *The Association is also referred to as the 'Glasgow Medical Association' in twentieth century sources.

Objects

To promote the campaign for national medical reform.

Membership

No details.

Meetings

F.U.

Publications

N.I.

Records

N.L.

Secondary References

Little (1932), 35.
McMenemy (1959), 186, 213, 218.
Stirling Journal and Advertiser 26 June 1840, 4.
Waddington (1984), 72.

135. Western Medical Club (1845–extant)

History

This social club seeks to promote social contact between medical practitioners from Glasgow and the surrounding country areas. Initially, social contact was maintained through two meetings per year. Members met for a dinner in Glasgow in the winter. This dinner often took place in the Hall of the Faculty of Physicians and Surgeons of Glasgow. In the summer, usually in July, the Club travelled to the country, frequently chartering a steamer to sail on the Clyde, on which dinner was served. The Club's dinners were partly financed through the members' subscriptions and the levying of fines for non-attendance at meetings. The average attendance at the Club's meetings between 1845–89 was thirty members. The Club celebrated its jubilee in Tarbet in 1895. Sir Thomas McCall Anderson, Regius Professor of Medicine at Glasgow University and Physician at Glasgow Western Infirmary, was for many years Secretary of the Club, he died in 1908.

Objects

To provide friendly and social intercourse between members of the medical profession in Glasgow and the West of Scotland.

Membership

Ten original members. Fifty-five in 1866. The Club had a limit placed on the size of its membership, in 1888 this was set at sixty, with thirty members each from Glasgow and the surrounding areas.

Meetings

Twice annually, once in Glasgow and once in the country.

Publications

N.I.

Records

N.L. See Library Royal College of Physicians and Surgeons of Glasgow, Miscellaneous Records, RCPSG 1/11/111, notes made by J. Finlayson on attendance, dates and places of meetings etc, while President of the Western Medical Club (1889).

Secondary References
Christie (1888), 186–8.
Walker Downie (1923), 87.
Duncan (1896), 198.
Gibson (1912), 276.

II

Alphabetical List of Scottish Student and Graduate Medical Societies

1. Aberdeen Medical Society* (1789–extant*)

History

This Society, which after 1811 became known as the Aberdeen-Medico Chirurgical Society (see entry 4 in main list), was until 1812, solely a student medical society. After this period of reorganisation, the Society was divided into senior and junior sections (also known as the first and second class). The latter consisted of student members, who elected their own office bearers, kept separate minutes, and held their meetings independently of the senior section, although on occasion the junior members were admitted to individual meetings of the senior section. The junior section had a chequered history. In 1821 its members were refused access to the Society's impressive library because of acts of vandalism on parts of the collection. More significantly, the student members of the Society became involved in resurrectionism, removing bodies from local church yards at night and bringing them to the Society's anatomical theatre for dissection. In 1806, the discovery of such a body illegally removed from a burial ground led to the members of the Society being taken before the Sheriff and a fine imposed. Undeterred, student members of the Society continued their resurrectionist exploits in 1818, and again in 1828. Despite such periods of activity, the junior section of the Society functioned intermittently, its separate minute books were discontinued and it ceased to exist in 1874, although the Society as a whole continues to the present.

Objects

To read papers on medical and scientific subjects.

Membership

Founded with twelve members. Membership fee was one guinea annually, raised to two guineas in 1868.

Meetings

Originally weekly, for a time after 1812 meetings were twice weekly on Tuesdays and Saturdays, by 1853 they were fortnightly, and by 1868 meetings were monthly.

Publications

Regulations of the Aberdeen Medico-Chirurgical Society with a List of members. (Aberdeen, 1833).

Records

Minute books of the Aberdeen Medical Society, and the junior section of the Aberdeen Medico-Chirurgical Society in the Library of the Aberdeen Medico-Chirurgical Society, Society Hall, Foresterhill, Aberdeen.

Secondary References

Craig, 'Aberdeen Medico-Chirurgical Society' (1937), 302–5.

Craig (1968), 5, 13.
Rodger (1893), *passim.*
Milne (1989), *passim.*
Riddell (1922), *passim.*
See also *Med.Dir.* and *Year-Book passim*

2. Aberdeen University Medical Students' Society (1864–extant)

History

This Society was formed shortly after the union of King's and Marischal Colleges as the University of Aberdeen in 1860, an event which increased the educational and social opportunities of medical students in the city. In 1872, a humorous publication entitled the *Aberdeen Medical Shaver* appeared, and this was followed in the 1872–3 session by the *Aberdeen Medical Student*, however, it is not clear if these publications were linked to the student Medical Society. The student Society originally met in the University, but in 1878, the Society wrote to the Aberdeen Medico-Chirurgical Society (entry 4 in main list) asking permission to hold meetings and scientific lectures in the latter Society's Hall, and this permission was granted. The Society had a chequered early existence, with several periods of inertia before it was placed on a more permanent footing in 1887, according to *Alma Mater* the Aberdeen University student magazine at the time. In 1922, almost fifty members of the student society attended a general meeting of the Medico-Chirurgical Society and several contributed to a discussion on the subject of the secrecy section of the Hippocratic Oath. There was also a Women's Medical Society set up at Aberdeen University sometime after the admission of female students in 1892, but there are no further details available on it.

Objects

To hold meetings, hear discussions and conduct experiments.

Membership

Open to students of medicine at Aberdeen University. Over fifty members in 1922.

Meetings

Fortnightly on Fridays at 7 p.m. on the University. After 1878 held monthly on Saturdays.

Publications

N.I.

Records

Minute books held by Aberdeen University Medical Students' Society. See also Aberdeen Medico-Chirurgical Society minute book, 10 and 17 January 1878; 19 January 1922.

Secondary References

Anderson (1988), 20, 33–4, 60.
Alma Mater 5 (1887–8), 18–19.
Ed.Al. (Aberdeen and Aberdeenshire suppl.), (1867), 42.
Med.Dir. (1868), 755.
Riddell (1922), 69.

3. American Medical Society (<1792–?)

History

One of many apparently short-lived student medical societies which flourished in Edinburgh in the last three decades of the eighteenth century, the American Medical like its similarly titled counterpart, the American Physical (4), sought to provide the numerous North American students who came to study medicine at Edinburgh a focus for debate and social intercourse. Little is known of this Society other than it held regular meetings during 1792. It is possible that the American Medical Society was amalgamated with the American Physical Society, which had a longer existence.

Objects

To provide a friendly forum for debate among American medical students.

Membership

Open to medical students from the American colonies studying at Edinburgh University.

Meetings

F.U.

Publications

N.I.

Records

N.L.

Secondary References

Johnston (1792), 48.
McElroy (1952), 305n.
Rosner (1991), 121.
Stroud (1820), xlvii

4. American Physical Society (<1790–6*)

History

In January 1790, the Society, in conjunction with the Royal Physical (21 and also see 51 in main list) and Hibernian Medical (16) Societies, presented an address to William Cullen, Professor of the Practice of Medicine, on his being honoured by the Edinburgh Town Council and the staff and students of Edinburgh University. Samples of the discussions of the American Physical Society, survive in a bound volume of dissertations on medical subjects covering the period 1794–6, some of which were delivered by Scottish and Irish, as well as American, students. *The Society was amalgamated with the Royal Physical Society in 1796, one of many smaller, less stable, societies to do so in the final years of the eighteenth century.

Objects

To provide educational facilities and occasional home atmosphere for American medical students in Edinburgh.

Membership

Membership predominantly, but not exclusively, American. The Society had twenty-nine members on its amalgamation with the Royal Physical Society in 1796.

Meetings

F.U.

Publications

N.I.

Records

One volume of dissertations covering the academic sessions 1794/5–1796/7 in Special Collections, Edinburgh University Library.

Secondary References

Comrie (1927), 215.

Edinburgh Magazine or Literary Miscellany 11 (1790), 9–10.
Finlayson (1956–8), 15.
McElroy (1952), 306.

5. Brown's Square Medical and Surgical Society (1826–7)

History

This Society, which originally met under the title of the Brown's Square Emulation Society, was formed by seven medical students to discuss cases arising in their work at Brown's Square Dispensary, Edinburgh. The Society met for less than a year.

Objects

'... to discuss cases of special interest met with in their [Dispensary] practice'. (Finlayson, (1956–8), 15)

Membership

The Society had seven members.

Meetings

F.U.

Publications

N.I.

Records

Brief minutes for the period August 1826–May 1827 along with laws and lists of members, in Special Collections, Edinburgh University Library.

Secondary References

Finlayson (1956–8), 15

6. Bute Medical Society (1915–extant)

History

The Society was founded by a group of six students, three male and three female, who had enrolled in medicine in 1914 at United College, University of St. Andrews. Though it began as a small society, due to the limited number of medical students enrolled at St. Andrews, it has remained flourishing to the present day. The Society was named after the Marquis of Bute, Rector of the University between 1892 and 1898, financer of the Bute Medical Building at United College, and founder of the Bute Chair of Anatomy in 1900. The Society has retained a strong social element, initially providing morning tea and coffee for its members, and holding a ball in the Martinmas term, as well as a continued involvement in charity fund raising.

Objects

'To provide lectures on clinical subjects to otherwise isolated pre-clinical medical students at [St. Andrews] ...' (Blair, 1987)

Membership

Open to students taking medical subjects at St. Andrews. Formed with six founder members. The various pre-clinical Professors were in turn elected as Honorary Presidents of the Society.

Meetings

Lectures are given before the Society every two months, approximately six meetings per academic session are held.

Publications

N.I.

Records

Early minutes of Society no longer extant. Remaining post-Second World War minutes held by Bute Medical Society, Bute Medical Building, University of St. Andrews.

Secondary References

Blair (1987), 188–9

7. Chirurgo Medical Society (1767–82*)

History

The Society was formed by students of medicine and surgery at Edinburgh University. The Society lapsed in 1771, but was reformed and remodelled in 1774. Ordinary members of the Chirurgo-Medical Society were obliged to read a dissertation before the Society in order of seniority. The Society exacted fines from its members, including a fine of five shillings to be levied on any member who disparaged the character of any of the medical professors of the University. *The Society amalgamated with the Royal Physical Society in 1782 (21 and also 51 in main list).

Objects

To hear dissertations on medical subjects.

Membership

The Society had two classes of membership, Ordinary and Honorary. The latter was open to members of the University medical faculty, Doctors of Medicine, and established surgeons.

Meetings

F.U.

Publications

N.I.

Records

One volume of Laws and Regulations from 1774, and another containing dissertations from 1780/1 in Special Collections, Edinburgh University Library.

Secondary References

Finlayson (1956–8), 15
McElroy (1952), 302
McElroy (1969), 136

8. Chirurgo–Obstetrical Society (1786–1792>)

History

John Aitken, a Fellow of the Royal College of Surgeons, was the driving force behind the Society, which met regularly for at least six years. Like many student societies in this period, it elected four Presidents annually, in order to lessen the burden of attendance of office bearers at every meeting. The inclusion of 'obstetrical' in the title of the society is noteworthy since midwifery enjoyed a less high reputation than other medical and surgical subjects and was the only course taught by the Edinburgh medical faculty not necessary for graduation.

Objects

Unknown.

Membership
No details as to size of membership.

Meetings
F.U.

Publications
John Aitken *An Address to the Chirurgo–Obstetrical Society: Delivered at their first meeting* (Edinburgh, 1786).

Records
N.L.

Secondary References
Ed. Al. (1787), n.p.
Johnston (1792), 48.
McElroy (1952), 305n.
Rosner (1991), 121.
Stroud (1820), xlvii.

9. Chirurgo–Physical Society (1788–96*)

History
This Society was yet another of the many student medical societies which flourished in Edinburgh in the last years of the eighteenth century. One volume of dissertations of members of the society covering the period 1789–91 is in existence, and includes two dissertations by the explorer, Mungo Park, on taenia and scurvy. *The Society, after a brief attempt to continue its existence through union with the American Physical Society (4), was united with the Royal Physical Society (21 and also see 51 in main list) in 1792.

Objects
To discuss the different branches of medicine.

Membership
No details available.

Meetings
F.U.

Publications
N.I.

Records
One volume of dissertations for 1789–91 in Special Collections, Edinburgh University Library.

Secondary References
Comrie (1927), 215.
Finlayson (1956–8), 16.
Glasgow Courier, 29 November 1791; December? 1792; January? 1794
Johnson (1792), 48
McElroy (1952), 304–5.
Rosner (1991), 121.

10. Dental Students' Association of Glasgow* (1880–extant)

History
*The Association subsequently changed its title to the Glasgow Dental Students' Society.

Meetings of the Association of Glasgow Dental Students were held in the newly opened Dental Hospital and School, which had been set up within Anderson's College to provide clinical teaching facilities in dental surgery in 1879 after the passage of the Dentists' Act. The arrangement with Anderson's College proved to be a short-term one, and an independent dental hospital and school for Glasgow was opened in 1885 in the city's George Square. The Dental Hospital and School is now situated in Sauchiehall Street, where Society meetings continue to be held. In the academic session 1979–80 the Dental Society celebrated its centenary. Meetings of the Society continue as a mixture of academic and social activities.

Objects

To represent dental students in matters affecting their interests, and to organise student activities in the Dental Hospital.

Membership

The Association enrolled thirty members in 1880.

Meetings

Monthly meetings and an annual dinner.

Publications

N.I.

Records

Minute books held by the Glasgow Dental Students' Society.

Secondary References

Brown (1960), 9.
British Journal of Dental Science, passim.
Glasgow University Student's Handbook 1963/64 , 122–23 and *passim.*

11. Edinburgh Medical Students Christian Association (<1887–?)

History

Reference to the existence of this Association was made in the obituary of William Brown, formerly President of the Royal College of Surgeons of Edinburgh, and Medical Officer at New Town Dispensary in 1887. Brown studied medicine at Edinburgh about 1815, and while at the University he felt a lack of Christian fellowship among his student colleagues. This was in contrast to the position by 1887, when the Medical Students' Christian Association was in a thriving condition. The Association may have been linked to the Edinburgh Medical Missionary Society (37 in main list), which sought to provide trained medical staff to work in overseas Christian missions, although there is no direct evidence of such a link.

Objects

No details.

Membership

The Association had over 200 members in 1887.

Meetings

F.U.

Publications

N.I.

Records

N.L.

Secondary References
EMJ 32/2 (January–June 1887), 765.

12. Edinburgh University Physiological Society (1904–13>)

History

The Society met in the Hughes Bennett classroom at Edinburgh University. In 1910, the Society held a joint meeting with the Royal Medical Society (22) to debate the issue, '... that the teaching of physiology in the University of Edinburgh is too much that of a pure science and has too little bearing on practical medicine'. John Tait, Secretary of the Physiological Society, and a member of staff in the University Physiology Laboratory, moved a negative motion and the original motion was defeated. President of the Society in 1908 was Sir Edward Albert Schaeffer, Professor of Physiology at Edinburgh University.

Objects

To hear papers and discussions on physiology and related scientific subjects.

Membership

Open to students and recent graduates of Edinburgh University. Staff of the University Physiology department were also members.

Meetings

On alternate Thursdays at 8 p.m. Annual meeting on the first Thursday in October.

Publications

N.I.

Records

N.L. See Royal Medical Society minute book, 21 January 1910, Society library, 22 Bristo Square, University of Edinburgh.

Secondary References
Med.Dir. (1908), 1368.

13. Edinburgh Women's Medical Society* (1913–52*)

History

From 1886 female medical students in Edinburgh were catered for at the Extra-Mural Edinburgh School of Medicine for Women established by Sophia Jex-Blake (physician at the Edinburgh Provident Dispensary for Women), and after 1894 Edinburgh University admitted female students for examination for degrees in Medicine. This decision led to the creation of the Medical College for Women, Edinburgh, but it was not until 1916 that female students were granted admission to the medical faculty of the University of Edinburgh. *The University Women's Medical Society, not to be confused with the Edinburgh Women's Medical Club (see entry 111 in main list), met in the University Women Students' Union. The fortnightly meetings were often addressed by guest medical speakers, although there were also clinical presentations, some by the members themselves. The Society continued to meet during the First World War, and in June 1915, Helen MacDougall, a former President of the Society gave an account of her experiences at the Scottish Women's Hospital at Kragujevicz, Serbia, which included a slide presentation. In 1916, the first meeting of the session in October was taken up by a discussion on issues arising from the admission of women to the Medical Faculty at Edinburgh University. In January 1920 the Society staged the first in a series of 'At Homes' for members and medical women in Edinburgh, which was attended by around 100 members and twenty-five female medical practitioners. In 1921, a reception was held by the Society for members of the Scottish Eastern Branch of the Medical Women's Federation. In the 1930s, the Edinburgh Society held a joint annual meeting with Glasgow University Queen Margaret Medical Club (22), each group acting as host in turn to the other. *No meetings of the Society were held after 1952, although it was not formally ended until 1957.

Objects

'To promote interest in and discussion of medical subjects. To foster corporate life and social intercourse among women medical undergraduates and graduates'. (Constitution of the Edinburgh Women's Medical Society, 1924)

Membership

The Society had forty-five members in 1939/40. Annual subscription was originally one shilling and sixpence, raised to two shillings and sixpence in 1919.

Meetings

Fortnightly.

Publications

N.I.

Records

Minute books for 1913–24, committee minute book, 1914–33, and account book for 1922–52, in Special Collections, Edinburgh University Library.

Secondary References

N.I.

14. Glasgow University Medico-Chirurgical Society (1802–extant)

History

The Glasgow University Medico-Chirurgical Society is the oldest existing medical society in Glasgow. Meetings of the Society were structured around the reading of dissertations by members, a synopsis of which had to be submitted a week before the meeting in question, followed by a discussion of the paper begun by a pre-designated 'leader of the discussion'. Fines were levied on members who failed to deliver their dissertations or lead the discussion as allocated; in 1868 these fines stood at two shillings and sixpence. The Society meets in the first two terms of the University's session, Martinmas and Candlemas. The Society maintained a library for many years, latterly held in the University Reading Room. Early in the twentieth century the Society began to hold regular clinical and demonstration nights. Meetings of the Society were disrupted, but not completely suspended, during the First World War, although several members of the Society left University to join the armed forces. In the 1920s, the Society in conjunction with the Glasgow female medical students' Queen Margaret Medical Club (22), held a regular annual outing to Bridge of Weir to visit various medical establishments in the area, rounded off by games and a dinner. Members of the female student medical society were invited to meetings of the Medico-Chirurgical Society on a regular basis after 1916, but were not admitted as members of the Society until 1969. The Society remains flourishing despite the rapid turnover in members common to all student societies. Over the years the Society has had many notable Honourary Presidents, including Sir Joseph Lister in 1892. Since 1934, the Society has published *Surgo*, a magazine for medical students at Glasgow University, which appears once a term.

Objects

'Mutual instruction of Members in matters of Medical Science'. (MS rules of Society 1862/3 held among papers of Society)

Membership

Open to male medical students and medical graduates of Glasgow University until 1969 when female medical students were granted admission. The Society had members in session 1867/8, 143 in 1914, 102 in 1918, 297 in 1927, 524 in 1959. Annual subscription to the Society remained nominal, two shillings and sixpence in 1870, one shilling in 1893, and three shillings and sixpence in 1963. It now stands at £20 for life membership.

Meetings

Weekly on various days throughout the Society's history to date.

Publications

Surgo (Glasgow, 1934–).
G.H. Eddington, *Medical Education* (Honorary Presidential Address, Nov. 4 1926) (Glasgow, 1927).

Records

Minute books from 1868 onwards, and other MS papers in the Archives Department, University of Glasgow.

Secondary References

Bowman (1942), 302, 360.
Walker Downie (1908), 2.
Kerr (1938), 88.
Year-Book (1886), 224.
Glasgow University Students' Handbook (1893), 99 and *passim*.

15. Glasgow University '88 Medical Club (1894–1907)

History

This Club is included in the 'Students' Societies Section' of medical societies, although it was in fact a graduates' association. Unlike the Edinburgh-based Octogenarian Club (20), this Club was restricted to medical graduates of a single University, Glasgow, and continued to hold its dinners in the University and to maintain an entry in the *Students' Handbook*. Membership of the Club was restricted to medical students enrolled at Glasgow University between 1884 and 1888. Although the Club was only convened once in every three years for dinner, contact was maintained by post in the intervening period, and indeed, a feature of the dinners was a statistical report on the fate of the original members of the society, e.g. in 1902 it was reported that 9 per cent of members had died since 1894, and over 14 per cent of the remainder lived abroad. Also, in the three years since the last dinner (1899), 10 per cent of all members had changed address. The final dinner of the Club was held in 1905, when it was reported that 11 per cent of the original membership had died, and although office-bearers were elected for the following three years, it was perhaps the effect of the ageing process on the Club's members which led to its cessation before the 1908 dinner was convened.

Objects

'... [to] encourag[e]... social intercourse among those who studied medicine at Glasgow in the years 1884–1888' (*Students' Handbook*, 1903/4)

Membership

Formed with 189 members in 1894. This had fallen to 168 in 1905.

Meetings

The Club held a dinner every three years.

Publications

N.I.

Records

N.L.

Secondary Sources

Glasgow University Students' Handbook, 1903/4, 89 and *passim*.

16. Hibernian Medical Society (<1790–9*)

History

The earliest notice of this Society comes from January 1790 when it presented a memorial address to Professor William Cullen, in conjunction with the Royal Physical (21 and also see 51 in main list) and American Physical (4) Societies. Not all dissertations read before the Society were on medical topics, others were on scientific, historical, and educational subjects. *In 1799, the Hibernian Medical Society united with the Royal Physical Society. The Society had over thirty members at the time of its union with the larger Society, which suggests that the prestige of the Royal Physical was increasing to the extent that it amalgamated larger and longer-lived student medical and scientific societies, as well as those in danger of extinction.

Objects

To provide educational and social facilities for Irish medical students studying at Edinburgh University.

Membership

Thirty-four members in 1799.

Meetings

F.U.

Publications

N.I.

Records

One volume of dissertations for 1798–9 in Special Collections, Edinburgh University Library.

Secondary References

Finlayson (1956–8), 16.
McElroy (1952), 306.
McElroy (1969), 138.

17. Hibernian Physical Society* (<1792–?)

History

Little is known of this Society of Irish medical students studying medicine at Edinburgh University, other than it met frequently during 1792. The Society was one of the many short-lived societies of medical students set up in Edinburgh in the final decades of the eighteenth century. It is possible that there was a link between this Society and the Hibernian Medical Society (16), or that they were rival organisations, but there is no firm evidence for either suggestion.

Objects

No details.

Membership

Open to Irish medical students studying at Edinburgh University.

Meetings
F.U.
Publications
N.I.
Records
N.L.
Secondary References
Johnson (1792), 48.
McElroy (1952), 305n.
Rosner (1991), 121.
Stroud (1820), xlvii.

18. Hunterian Medical Society (1824–68)

History

The Hunterian Medical Society was one of the Associated Societies of the University of Edinburgh, as for a time was the Royal Physical Society (21 and entry 51 in main list). The Associated Societies met in their own hall at the University on different evenings of the week. The Society possessed its own library which amounted to 500 volumes in 1834. The Hunterian Medical Society levied a great many fines on recalcitrant members; including a fine of five shillings for failure to read an essay as promised, and a fine of two shillings and sixpence for writing a false address in the Librarian's loans book. After 1834, the Society provided two silver medal prizes worth two guineas each for the best paper read and the best debater in the Society. These prizes were awarded after a ballot among the members. A long-term member of the Society was Peter David Handyside, Surgeon at the Royal Infirmary and Extra-Mural Lecturer in Anatomy. He was the Society's final Treasurer.

Objects

'... the cultivation of medicine and the auxiliary sciences'. (*Medical Directory*, 1853)

Membership

Founded with eight members in 1824. The Society had thirty-three members in 1858, and twenty-four at its cessation in 1868. The original annual subscription was one guinea, although this had been reduced to seven shillings and sixpence by 1868.

Meetings

Weekly at 8 p.m. on Fridays during the University Session.

Publications

The Hunterian Medical Society's Library (Edinburgh, 1834).
The Laws of the Hunterian Medical Society of Edinburgh (Edinburgh, 1840).

Records

Minute books for 1842–50 and 1855–68, cash book and other papers in Special Collections, Edinburgh University Library.

Secondary References

Ed.Al. (1829), 334 and *passim*.
Finlayson (1956–58), 16.
Med.Dir., (1853), 783–4.

19. Medical Society of Aberdeen (<1768–71?)

History

This small society was a short-lived precursor of the Aberdeen Medical Society (1), set up by James Clark, a physician, during his student days. Although well attended during his time at Marischal College, it ended soon after his departure.

Objects

To hear papers and discuss medical and scientific subjects.

Membership

Had a small group of members, but no specific details as to numbers.

Meetings

F.U.

Publications

N.I.

Records

N.L.

Secondary References

Riddell (1922), 12–13.

20. Octogenarian Club (1895–1939)

History

This social medical Club was formed at a meeting of five practitioners in the Royal College of Physicians in Edinburgh. Membership of the Club was limited to medical graduates from the years 1880 to 1889, hence the Club's somewhat unusual title. The Presidency was to be held in rotation by order of seniority, and was to be decided alphabetically in the case of members who had graduated in the same year. The light-hearted nature of the Octogenarian Club is evident from the fact that the President's annual oration was to be on a non-medical subject not exceeding ten minutes in length. Among the founder members of the Club were Dairmid Noel Paton, Lecturer in the Institutes of Medicine at Edinburgh University, and Norman Walker, Assistant Physician in Dermatology at Edinburgh Royal Infirmary. One of the Club's specialities was a jocular customised menu for the Winter dinner; in 1896, the menu was printed as a series of advertisements for patent medicines, written as caricatures of the Club's member's, and in 1902, was written up as a casebook, for the 'Octogenarian ward'. The Club's festivities were suspended during the First World War, and during the course of the nineteen-thirties the Club became less vigorous as members grew older and died. In particular, the golf tournaments which were held at summer meetings of the Club were less keenly contested. No winter meeting of the Club was held in November 1939 due to 'present conditions', and the Club was never re-formed.

Objects

To maintain social contacts between medical graduates who qualified during the 1880s.

Membership

Originally limited to twenty members, the total number of members was forty-four. Admission by ballot on the recommendation of the committee. Annual subscription was one guinea.

Meetings

Twice a year in November and May.

Publications

N.I.

Records

Minute books and other records, including photographic portraits of members, in the Royal College of Physicians Library, Edinburgh.

Secondary References

N.I.

21. Physico-Chirurgical Society* (1774–extant*)

History

*The Society shortened its title to the Physical Society in 1780, and in 1782 it amalgamated with the Chirurgo Medical Society (7) to become what was known after 1788 as the Royal Physical Society (51 in main list). Members of the Society were free to challenge the activities of office-bearers of the Society, but if the office-bearer were exonerated from the charge of misconduct, the accusing member was liable to a fine equal to that originally called for of the office-bearer; this was increased to a fine of ten shillings and sixpence when a member had called for the deposition of an office-bearer for misconduct. Ordinary members of the Society read dissertations in order of seniority, these were to be prepared two weeks before they were delivered, in order that they could be circulated among other members. Failure to prepare dissertations in advance resulted in a fine against the recalcitrant member, hence dissertations read before the Society were invariably methodical, with a strong medico-scientific content. The original Society had two levels of membership, Ordinary and Honorary, with the latter reserved for prominent members of the local profession and men of international repute, including Benjamin Franklin and John Adams, both future Presidents of the United States.

Objects

The cultivation of physical sciences.

Membership

Established with eighteen founder members, the Society soon grew in size. It had 440 members in 1788, 1300 in 1830, and 1600 in 1853. Membership fee was £1/5 shillings in 1853.

Meetings

Weekly on Tuesdays at 8 p.m. during the Winter session of the University of Edinburgh.

Publications

Laws and Regulations of the Physical Society instituted at Edinburgh July 2 1771 (Edinburgh, 1780).

Records

Four volumes of dissertations from the years 1775–80 are held in Special Collections, Edinburgh University Library.

Secondary References

Comrie (1927), 215.
Finlayson (1956–8), 17.
Johnson (1792), 48.
McElroy (1952), 302.
McElroy (1969).
Proceedings of the Royal Physical Society 4 (1874–8), 7.
Rosner (1991), 121.

22. Queen Margaret College Medical Society* (1893–1969*)

History

*The Society became known as the Queen Margaret Medical Club shortly after its foundation. The Society was established to help counteract the segregation of female from male medical students both in terms of teaching and also in their long-term exclusion from the male-only Glasgow University Medico-Chirurgical Society (15). This latter exclusion was finally ended when the two organisations merged in 1969, although there had been occasional joint meetings of the Societies within ten years of the admission of women medical students to Queen Margaret College in 1898. Female medical students represented a sizeable proportion of all female students at the University of Glasgow at the beginning of the twentieth century. In session 1902/3 there were eighty female medical students among a total of 360 female students at the University. Meetings of the Queen Margaret Medical Society consisted of lectures given before the Society by guest speakers, plus the presentation and discussion of papers by members. Later in the twentieth century, clinical demonstrations around the various teaching hospitals in Glasgow were held on a weekly basis, while lectures were restricted to two annual addresses before the Society by prominent guest speakers. In the 1930s, the Club held joint annual meetings with the Edinburgh Women's Medical Society (13).

Objects

To encourage and further the interests of female medical students at Glasgow University.

Membership

Open to all female medical students and female medical graduates of the University.

Meetings

Originally held weekly on Tuesdays.

Publications

The Club's affairs were recorded in *Surgo*, the magazine for Glasgow University medical students established in 1934.

Records

N.L. See Glasgow University Medico-Chirurgical Society minute book, 15 March 1916, and *passim*.

Secondary References

Glasgow University Students' Handbook, 1939/40, 143 and *passim*.

23. Royal Medical Society (1737–extant)

History

Although formally constituted in 1737 as the Medical Society, there had been informal meetings of a group of six medical students since 1734. The Society was founded with ten members, who presented a discourse on a medical subject of their choice before the other members. Later meetings included discussion of specific medical and surgical cases. Initially, the Society met in local taverns in Edinburgh, but after 1763, the Society met in the Royal Infirmary, until sufficient funds were raised for the erection of the Society's own premises in 1776. The opening of this building allowed for the expansion of the Society's library, as well as providing a hall for meetings and rooms for experiments to be carried out. The Society was given a further boost to its prestige in 1778, when it was granted a Royal Charter by George III. In 1784, the Society inaugurated a Prize essay competition on medical and related subjects; the annual prize offered was a gold medal worth twenty guineas. Towards the end of the eighteenth century, the Society published three volumes of inaugural dissertations read by students in the Edinburgh Medical

School under the title of *Thesaurus Medicus*. Also in the early 1780s, the Society went through a difficult period owing to the controversy over the Brunonian system of medicine which found both supporters and opponents in the ranks of the Society (John Brown had been President of the Society on three occasions), and led to resignations among Society members. In 1823, Andrew Combe's dissertation before the Society on Phrenology attracted a crowd of 400 to the meeting, and prompted a discussion which lasted until the early hours of the morning. In 1868, the Society was addressed by John Hughes Bennett, Professor of the Institutes of Medicine and Clinical Medicine at Edinburgh University. Since 1871, an eminent medical figure has been invited to deliver an annual inaugural address before the Society. In the course of the twentieth century, the Society began to hold clinical meetings and arrange film shows on medical subjects, in addition to its regular meetings.

Objects

'The advancement of Medical Science, and the discussion of questions either purely medical or akin to Medicine'. (Hume (1853), 169)

Membership

Members admitted on the recommendation of six existing members. Initial membership costs were sixpence per week. In 1884, membership was 120, and the annual subscription was two guineas. The subscription fee remained at this level until the 1960s. In 1951, the Society had 200 members.

Meetings

Weekly, initially on Saturdays, later this was changed to Fridays, during the Society's session of the first two academic terms.

Publications

Andrew Duncan, *A Short Account of the Commencement, Progress, and Present State of the Buildings Belonging to the Royal Medical Society of Edinburgh* (Edinburgh, 1819).
Gray (1952).
Stroud (1820).
Thesaurus Medicus (Edinburgh, 1778–85)

Records

Minute books, membership lists and other records in the library of the Royal Medical Society, 22 Bristo Square, University of Edinburgh.

Secondary References

Comrie (1927), 214–16.
Edinburgh University Journal 33 (1988), 109–11.
Finlayson (1956–8), 18.
Hume (1853), 169–70.
Johnson (1792), 48–53.
Lawrence (1984), 200–17, and *passim*.
McElroy (1952), 363–74 and *passim*.
McElroy (1969), 131–4.
Rosner (1991), 119–34.
See also *EMSJ, EMJ, Med.Dir.* and *Year-Book, passim*.

24. St. Andrews University Medical Society (1916–?)

History

The Society was formed in University College in the Autumn of 1916, perhaps to counter the attractions of the United College rival, the Bute Medical Society (6), which was set up in 1915. The first President of the Society was Margaret Shirlaw (later

Menzies Campbell), who qualified in 1918 and later became House Surgeon at Doncaster Royal Infirmary. The first lecture before the Society was given by Alexander Mitchell Stalker, Professor of Medicine at the University, and Physician at Dundee Royal Infirmary. There is no indication as to the duration or the ultimate fate of the Society.

Objects

To provide educational and social facilities for medical students at the University of St. Andrews.

Membership

No details as to size.

Meetings

F.U.

Publications

N.I.

Records

N.L.

Secondary References

Blair (1987), 188.

25. St Mungo's College Medical Society (1878–1914>)

History

The Society was intended to serve the further educational and social interests of the medical students enrolled at St. Mungo's extra mural medical school in Glasgow (also known as the Royal Infirmary medical school) which had been set up in 1876. The Society possessed its own library of medical works. In 1893, the Honorary President of the Society was James Stirton, Lecturer in Midwifery at the College, and in 1898 this office was held by Francis Horatio Napier, Professor of Ophthalmology at the College, and Ophthalmic Surgeon at Glasgow Royal Infirmary. The Society may have come to an end during the First World War, although the College itself continued until 1945 when extra-mural medical schools were abolished in favour of concentration on University medical teaching.

Objects

To provide educational and social opportunities for medical students at St. Mungo's College.

Membership

Open to medical students enrolled at St. Mungo's College.

Meetings

Weekly at the College on Saturday mornings. Annual meeting in late October or in November.

Publications

N.I.

Records

N.L.

Secondary References

Med.Dir. (1893), 1371 and *passim.*

Bibliography

BOOKS*

Wendy Alexander, *First Ladies of Medicine* (Glasgow, 1987).
Mabel D. Allardyce, *The Library of the Medico-Chirurgical Society of Aberdeen* (Aberdeen, 1934).
R. D. Anderson, *Education and Opportunity in Victorian Scotland: Schools and Universities* (Oxford, 1983).
——, *The Student Community at Aberdeen 1860-1939* (Aberdeen, 1988).
R. G. W. Anderson and A. D. C. Simpson, (eds), *Early Years of the Edinburgh Medical School* (Edinburgh, 1976).
J. Wallace Anderson, *Four Chiefs of the G. R. I.* (Glasgow, 1916).
Lady Frances Balfour, *Dr. Elsie Inglis* (1918).
Jonathan Barry and Colin Jones (eds), *Medicine and Charity before the Welfare State* (1991).
E. Moberley Bell, *Storming the Citadel: The Rise of the Woman Doctor* (1953).
J. S. G. Blair, *History of Medicine in St. Andrews University* (Edinburgh, 1987).
——, *Ten Tayside Doctors* (Edinburgh, 1990).
A. K. Bowman, *Life and Teaching of Sir Wiliam MacEwen* (1942).
Jeanne L. Brand, *Doctors and the State: The British Medical Profession and Government Action in Public Health, 1870-1912* (Baltimore, 1965).
James Bridie, *One Way of Living* (Glasgow, 1939).
John Malcolm Bulloch, *History of the University of Aberdeen 1495-1895* (Aberdeen, 1895).
W. F. Bynum and Roy Porter (eds), *William Hunter and the Eighteenth Century Medical World* (Cambridge, 1985).
——, *Brunonianism in Britain and Europe* (*Medical History* Supplement No. 8, 1988).
R. H. Campbell and Andrew S. Skinner (eds), *The Origins and Nature of the Scottish Enlightenment* (Edinburgh, 1982).
J. Menzies Campbell, *From a Trade to a Profession: Byways in Dental History* (Alva, 1958).
R. G. Cant, *The University of St. Andrews: A short history* (Edinburgh, 1946).
A. M. Carr-Saunders and P. A. Wilson, *The Professions* (Oxford, 1930).
Jennifer J. Carter and Joan H. Pittock (eds), *Aberdeen and the Enlightenment* (Aberdeen, 1987).
A. K. Chalmers, *The Health of Glasgow: An outline* (Glasgow, 1930).
Olive Checkland, *Philanthropy in Victorian Scotland* (Edinburgh, 1980).
—— and Margaret Lamb (eds), *Health Care as Social History: The Glasgow Case* (Aberdeen, 1982) .
John Chiene, *Looking Back: 1907-1860* (Edinburgh, 1908).

*Published in London unless otherwise stated.

James Christie, *The Medical Institutions of Glasgow* (2nd edn, Glasgow, 1888).

Sir Robert Christison, *The Life of Sir Robert Christison, Bart, edited by his sons* (2 vols, Edinburgh, 1885-6).

Sir Henry Thomas Cockburn, *Memorials of his Time* (Edinburgh, 1856, 2nd edn 1910).

——, *The Journal of Henry Thomas Cockburn* (2 vols, Edinburgh, 1874).

E. Colman (ed.), *The Scottish Paediatric Society, 1922-1972* (Glasgow, 1972).

George Combe, *Life and Correspondence of Andrew Combe* (Edinburgh, 1850).

John Comrie, *History of Scottish Medicine to 1860* (1927).

Roger Cooter, *The Cultural Meaning of Popular Science: Phrenology and the Organisation of Consent in Nineteenth Century Britain* (Cambridge, 1984).

——, *Phrenology in the British Isles: An Annotated, Historical Biobibliography and Index* (Metuchen, NJ, 1989).

William Stuart Craig, *History of the Royal College of Physicians of Edinburgh* (Edinburgh, 1926).

Clarendon Hyde Creswell, *The Royal College of Surgeons of Edinburgh: Historical Notes from 1505 to 1905* (Edinburgh, 1926).

Michael J. Cullen, *The Statistical Movement in Early Victorian Britain* (Hassocks, Sussex, 1975).

Robert Dingwall and Philip Lewis (eds), *The Sociology of the Professions* (1983).

Jean Donnison, *Midwives and Medical Men* (1977).

J. Dougall, *Historical Sketch of the Glasgow Southern Medical Society* (Glasgow, 1888).

Derek A. Dow, *The Royal Alexandria Infirmary and Allied Institutions 1786-1986* (Paisley, 1988).

Dow and Kenneth C. Calman (eds), *The Royal Medico-Chirurgical Society of Glasgow: A History, 1814-1989* (Glasgow, 1991).

Dow and Stefan Slater (eds), *The Victoria Infirmary of Glasgow 1890-1990: A Centenary History* (Glasgow, 1990).

J. Walker Downie, *The Early Physicians and Surgeons of the Western Infirmary, Glasgow* (Glasgow, 1923).

Alexander Duncan, *Memorials of the Faculty of Physicians and Surgeons of Glasgow 1599-1850* (Glasgow, 1896).

Norman R. Eder, *National Health Insurance and the medical Profession in Britain, 1913-1939* (New York, 1982).

Edinburgh Medical Society, *Medical Essays and Observations* (6 vols, 1733-39).

Edinburgh Philosophical Society, *Essays and Observations Physical and Literary* (Edinburgh, 1754, 1756, 1771).

Edinburgh Philosophical Society, *Proposals for the Regulation of a Society for Improving Arts and Sciences, and particularly, Natural Knowledge* (Edinburgh, 1737).

Owen Dudley Edwards, *Burke and Hare* (Edinburgh, 1977).

Phillip Elliott, *The Sociology of the Professions* (1972).

John Eyler, *Victorian Social Medicine* (Baltimore, 1979).

J. Ferrier, *Greenock Infirmary 1806-1968* (Greenock, 1968).

Eliot Friedson, *The Profession of Medicine* (New York, 1972).

John Fry (ed.), *Primary Care* (1980).

George Alexander Gibson, *Life of Sir William Tennant Gairdner* (1912).

Henry J. C. Gibson, *History of Dundee Royal Infirmary 1789-1948* (Dundee, 1948).

Thomas Gibson, *Royal College of Physicians and Surgeons of Glasgow* (Edinburgh, 1983).

Bentley B. Gilbert, *The Evolution of National Insurance in Great Britain: The Origins of the Welfare State* (1966).

Lindsay Granshaw and Roy Porter (eds), *The Hospital in History* (1989).

James Gray, *History of the Royal Medical Society of Edinburgh 1737-1937* (Edinburgh, 1952).

John Gregory, *Lectures on the Duties and Qualifications of a Physician* (1772).
David Hamilton, *The Healers: A History of Medicine in Scotland* (Edinburgh, 1981).
J. D. Hargreaves with A. Forbes, *Aberdeen University 1945-1981* (Aberdeen, 1989).
R. W. Harris, *National Health Insurance in Great Britain 1911-1946* (1946).
T. Brown Henderson, *The History of Glasgow Dental Hospital and School 1879-1959* (Glasgow, 1960).
Christine Hillam (ed.), *Roots of Dentistry* (1990).
S. W. F. Holloway, *The Royal Pharmaceutical Society of Great Britain 1841-1991* (1991).
Geoffrey Holmes, *Augustan England: Professions, Status and Society, 1680-1730* (1982).
Frank Honigsbaum, *The Division of British Medicine: a history of the separation of general practice from hospital care, 1911-1968* (1979).
David Bayne Horne, *A Short History of the University of Edinburgh* (Edinburgh, 1967).
Reverend A. Hume, *Learned Societies and Printing Clubs of the United Kingdom* (1853).
Thomas Hunt (ed.), *The Medical Society of London, 1773-1973* (1972).
Jamieson B. Hurry, *The Ideals and Organisation of a Medical Society* (1913).
G. Irving, *Dumfries and Galloway Royal Infirmary: The first two hundred years* (Dumfries, 1975).
L. S. Jacyna (ed.), *A Tale of Three Cities: The Correspondence of William Sharpey and Allen Thomson*, (*Medical History* Supplement No. 9, 1989).
J. Johnson, *A Guide for Gentlemen Studying Medicine at the University of Edinburgh* (1792).
Chauncey D. Leake (ed.), *Percival's Medical Ethics* (Baltimore, 1927).
R. A. B. Leaper (ed.), *Health, Wealth, and Housing* (Oxford, 1980).
H. F. Lechmere-Taylor, *A Century of Service 1841-1941: Edinburgh Medical Missionary Society* (Edinburgh, 1941).
J. M. Leighton, *Fife Illustrated* (vol. 2) (Cupar, 1840).
Ernest Muirhead Little (ed.), *History of the British Medical Association 1832-1932* (1932).
Henry Lonsdale, *A Sketch of the Life and Writings of Robert Knox* (1870).
Irvine Loudon, *Medical Care and the General Practitioner 1750-1950* (Oxford, 1986).
John Lowe, *Medical Missions: Their Place and Power* (1886).
D. McCrone *et al.* (eds), *The Making of Scotland: Nation, culture and social change* (Edinburgh, 1989).
Davis D. McElroy, *Scotland's Age of Improvement: A Survey of Eighteenth-Century Literary Clubs and Societies* (Washington, 1969).
J. McKendrick, *Annals of the Round Table Club* (Stonehaven, 1908).
Gordon McLachlan (ed.), *Improving the Commonweal: Aspects of Scottish Health Services 1900-1984* (Edinburgh, 1987).
William H. McMenemy, *The Life and Times of Sir Charles Hastings* (Edinburgh and London, 1959).
J. D. Mackie, *University of Glasgow 1451-1951* (Glasgow, 1954).
Rosalind K. Marshall, *Virgins and Viragos: A history of women in Scotland from 1680 to 1980* (1983).
Leslie G. Matthews, *History of Pharmacy in Britain* (Edinburgh, 1962).
Russell C. Maulitz, *Morbid Appearances: The Anatomy of Pathology in the Early 19th Century* (Cambridge/New York, 1987).
George P. Milne (ed.), *The Aberdeen Medico-Chirurgical Society: A Bicentennial History 1789-1989* (Aberdeen, 1989).
Sir Norman Moore and Stephen Paget, *The Royal Medical and Chirurgical Society of London: Centenary, 1805-1905* (Aberdeen, 1905).
Ornella Moscucci, *The Science of Woman: Gynaecology and Gender in England, 1800-1929* (Cambridge, 1990).
James Muir, *John Anderson and the College He Founded* (Glasgow, 1950).
Charles Newman, *Evolution of Medical Education in the Nineteenth Century* (1957).

Phillip A. Nicholls, *Homoeopathy and the Medical Profession* (1988).

C. D. O'Malley (ed.), *History of Medical Education* (Berkeley, CA, 1970).

Noel and José Parry, *The Rise of the Medical Profession: A Study of Collective Social Mobility* (1976).

Thomas Percival, *Medical Ethics ; or, a Code of Institutes and Precepts, Adapted to the Professional Conduct of Physicians and Surgeons* (2nd edn, 1827).

Harold Perkin, *The Rise of Professional Society: England since 1880* (1989).

M. Jeanne Peterson, *The Medical Profession in Mid-Victorian London* (Berkeley, CA, 1979).

N. T. Phillipson and Rosalind Mitchison, *Scotland in the Age of Improvement* (Edinburgh, 1970).

J. V. Pickstone, *Medicine and Industrial Society: A History of Hospital Development in Manchester and its Region, 1752-1946* (Manchester, 1985).

Sir D'Arcy Power (ed.), *British Medical Societies* (1939).

F. N. L. Poynter (ed.), *The Evolution of Medical Practice in Britain* (1961).

—— (ed.), *The Evolution of Medical Education in Britain* (1966).

Isobel Rae, *Knox, the Anatomist* (Edinburgh, 1964).

Records of the 'Aesculapian' (Edinburgh, 1888, with supplement, 1906).

W. J. Reader, *Professional Men* (1966).

Walter Rivington, *The Medical Profession* (Dublin, 1879).

George Gladstone Robertson, *Gorbals Doctor* (1970).

Ruth Richardson, *Death, Dissection and the Destitute* (1987).

John Scott Riddell, *Records of the Aberdeen Medico-Chirurgical Society from 1789 to 1922* (Aberdeen, 1922).

Guenter B. Risse, *Hospital Life in Enlightenment Scotland: Care and Teaching at the Royal Infirmary of Edinburgh* (Cambridge, 1986).

Ella Hill Burton Rodger, *Aberdeen Doctors at Home and Abroad: The Narrative of a Medical School* (Edinburgh, 1893).

Lisa Rosner, *Medical Education in the Age of Improvement* (Edinburgh, 1991).

Michael Sanderson, *Universities and British Industry* (1972).

Sanderson (ed.), *Universities in the Nineteenth Century* (1975).

Gareth Shaw and Allison Tipper (eds), *British Directories: A bibliographical guide to directories published in England and Wales (1850-1950) and Scotland (1773-1950)* (1988).

John A. Shepherd, *Simpson and Syme of Edinburgh* (Edinburgh, 1969).

Richard Harris Shyrock, *The Development of Modern Medicine* (Wisconsin, 1979).

Myrtle Simpson, *Simpson the Obstetrician* (1972).

Brian Abel-Smith, *The Hospitals 1800-1948* (1964).

F. B. Smith, *The People's Health 1830-1910* (New York 1979).

R. W. Innes Smith, *English-speaking Students at the University of Leyden* (Edinburgh, 1932).

Donald Southgate, *University Education in Dundee: A centenary history* (Edinburgh, 1982).

Rosemary Stevens, *Medical Practice in Modern England: The Impact of Specialisation and State Medicine* (1966).

Lawrence Stone (ed.), *The University and Society vol. 2: Europe, Scotland and the United States from the Eighteenth to the Twentieth Century* (1975).

John Strang, *Glasgow and its Clubs* (3rd edn, Glasgow, 1864).

William Stroud, *History of the Medical Society of Edinburgh* (Edinburgh, 1820).

W. J. Stuart, *History of the Aesculapian Club* (Edinburgh, 1949).

A. M. Wright Thomson, *History of the Glasgow Eye Infirmary 1824-1962* (Glasgow, 1963).

——, *History of the Scottish Opthalmological Club* (Edinburgh, 1979).

John L. Thornton, *Medical Books, Libraries and Collectors* (1949).
Margaret Todd, *Life of Sophia Jex-Blake* (1918).
A. Logan Turner (ed.), *History of the University of Edinburgh 1883-1933* (Edinburgh, 1933).
Logan Turner, *Story of a Great Hospital: The Royal Infirmary of Edinburgh* (Edinburgh, 1937).
H. Lewis Ulman (ed.), *Minutes of the Aberdeen Philosophical Society 1758-1773* (Aberdeen, 1991).
Paul Vaughan, *Doctors' Commons: A Short History of the British Medical Association* (1959).
Ivan Waddington, *The Medical Profession in the Industrial Revolution* (Dublin, 1984).
Roy Wallis (ed.), *On the Margins of Science* (Sociological Review Monograph, number 27) (Keele, 1979).
Mary Roth Walsh, *'Doctors Wanted: No Women Need Apply': Sexual Barriers in the Medical Profession 1835-1975* (New Haven, Conn., 1977).
Hewett Cottrell Watson, *Statistics of Phrenology: Being a Sketch of the Progress and Present State of that Science in the British Isles* (1836).
H. L. Watson-Wemyss, *Record of the Edinburgh Harveian Society* (Edinburgh, 1933).
John Woodward, *To do the Sick no Harm: A Study of the British Voluntary Hospital System to 1875* (1974).
Woodward and D. Richards (eds),. *Health Care and Popular Medicine in Nineteenth Century England* (1977).
Rex E. Wright-St. Clair, *Drs Monro: A Medical Saga* (1974) .
A. J. Youngson, *The Scientific Revolution in Victorian Medicine* (1979).

ARTICLES AND PAMPHLETS

A. Batty Shaw, 'The Oldest Medical Societies in Great Britain', *Medical History* 12 (1967), 232–44 .
Robert A. Bayliss, 'The Round Table Club, Edinburgh', *Practitioner* 224 (1980), 438–40.
J. Bishop, 'Medical Societies', *Chambers Encyclopaedia* (9th edn, 1950), 207–9.
——, 'Medical Book Societies in England in the 18th and 19th centuries', *Bulletin Medical Librarians Association,* 45 (1957), 337–50.
D. U. Bloor, 'The Rise of the General Practitioner in the Nineteenth Century', *J. Royal College of General Practitioners* 28 (1978), 288–91.
G. Cantor, 'Phrenology in Early Nineteenth Century Edinburgh: An Historiographical Discussion', *Annals of Science* 32 (1975), 195–218.
——, 'A Critique of Shapin's Social Interpretation of the Edinburgh Phrenology Debate', *Annals of Science* 33 (1975), 245–56.
Anand C. Chitnis, 'Medical Education in Edinburgh 1790-1826 and some Victorian Consequences', *Medical History* 17 (1973), 173–85.
J. R. R. Christie, 'Edinburgh Medicine in the Eighteenth century: The View from the Students', *Bull. Society Social History Medicine* 19 (1976), 13–15.
Adam Collier, 'Social Origins of a Sample of Entrants to Glasgow University', *Sociol. Review* 30 (1938), 161–85; 262–77.
John D. Comrie, 'The Edinburgh Harveian Society', *Medical Press and Circular* 195 (1937), 476–9.
John Craig, 'The Aberdeen Medico-Chirurgical Society', *Medical Press and Circular* 195 (1937), 302–5.
——, 'The Aberdeen Medico-Chirurgical Society', *Medical News* 9 August 1968, 5, 13.
J. K. Crellin, 'The Growth of Professionalism in Nineteenth Century Pharmacy', *Medical History* 11 (1967), 215–27.
M. Anne Crowther, 'Paupers of Patients?: Obstacles to Professionalism in the Poor Law

Medical Services before 1914', *J. History of Medicine and Allied Sciences* 60 (1984), 33–54.

H. J. H. Drummond, 'Early Medical and Scientific Societies of North East Scotland', *Bibliotheck* 1 (1956–58), 31–3.

——, 'Early Medical and Scientific Societies', *Library Association Record* 58 (1956), 243–4.

Marguerite W. Dupree and M. Anne Crowther, 'A Profile of the Medical Profession in Scotland in the Early Twentieth Century: The *Medical Directory* as a Historical Source', *Bull. Hist. Med.* 65 (1991), 209–33.

Roger L. Emerson, 'The Philosophical Society of Edinburgh 1737–1747', *Brit. J. History of Science* 12 (1979),151–91.

——, 'The Philosophical Society of Edinburgh 1748–1768', *Brit. J. History of Science* 14 (1981), 133–76.

——, 'The Philosophical Society of Edinburgh 1768–1783', *Brit. J. History of Science* 15 (1985), 255–303 .

——, 'The Scottish Enlightenment and the End of the Philosophical Society of Edinburgh', *Brit. J. History of Science* 21 (1988), 33–66.

——, 'Science and the Origins and Concerns of the Scottish Enlightenment', *History of Science* 26 (1988), 333–66.

——, 'Sir Robert Sibbald, Kt, the Royal Society of Scotland and the Origins of the Scottish Enlightenment', *Annals of Science* 45 (1988), 41–72.

H. D. Erlam, 'Alexander Monro, *primus*', *Edinburgh University Journal* 17 (1953–5), 77–105.

C. P. Finlayson, 'Records of Scientific and Medical Societies Preserved in the University Library, Edinburgh', *Bibliotheck* 1/3 (1956–8), 14–19.

Finlayson, 'Records of Scientific and Medical Societies preserved in the University Library Edinburgh: Additions', *Bibliotheck* 4 (1963–6), 38.

E. G. Forbes, 'The Professionalisation of Dentistry in the United Kingdom', *Medical History* 29 (1985), 169–81.

Daniel G. Gordon, 'Aberdeenshire Medical Associations', *Aberdeen PostGraduate Medical Bulletin* (October 1968), 3–5.

——, 'The Garioch and Northern Medical Association', *Aberdeen PostGraduate Medical Bulletin* (October 1970), 19–23.

Douglas Guthrie, 'The Aesculapian Club of Edinburgh', *Univ. of Edinb. Jnl* 23 (1967), 245–50.

——, 'The Harveian Tradition in Scotland', *J. of the History of Medicine and Allied Sciences* 12 (pt. 2) (1957), 120–5.

——, 'The Edinburgh Pathological Club', *Medical History* 10 (1966), 87–91.

Bernice Hamilton, 'The Medical Profession in the 18th century' *Economic History Review* [2nd series], 4 (1951), 141–69.

Peter Handyside, 'Valedictory Address to the Medico-Chirurgical Society of Edinburgh', *Edinburgh Medical Journal* 19/2 (1874), 769–87; 895–912; 1004–20; 1092–1105.

History of Science and Medicine Unit, Edinburgh *Scotland's Cultural Heritage vol 1: One Hundred Medical and Scientific Fellows of the Royal Society of Edinburgh, elected from 1782 to 1832* (Edinburgh, 1981) (pamphlet).

History of Science and Medicine Unit, Edinburgh, *Scotland's Cultural Heritage vol 3: The Royal Society of Edinburgh: One Hundred Medical Fellows elected from 1783–1844* (Edinburgh, 1982) (pamphlet).

Sydney W. F. Holloway, 'Medical Education in England, 1830–1858: A Sociological Analysis', *History* 49 (1964), 299–324.

——, 'The Apothecaries', Act 1815: A Reinterpretation – Part One: The Origins of the Act', *Medical History* 10 (1966), 107–29.

——, 'The Apothecaries Act 1815: A Reinterpretation – Part Two: The Consequences of the Act', *Medical History* 10 (1966), 221–36.

James Innes, 'The Harveians of Edinburgh: Their First Two Hundred Years', *Scottish Medical Journal* 28 (1983), 285–9.

Jacqueline Jenkinson, 'The Role of Medical Societies in the rise of the Scottish Medical Profession, 1730–1939', *Social History of Medicine* 4 (1991), 253–76.

Nicholas D. Jewson, 'Medical Knowledge and the Patronage System in Eighteenth-century England', *Sociology* 8 (1974), 369–85.

A. B. Kerr, 'The Royal Medico-Chirurgical Society of Glasgow', *Medical Press and Circular* 198 (1938), 83–97.

Christopher Lawrence, 'Incommunicable Knowledge: Science, Technology and the Clinical Art 1850–1914', *J. Contemporary History* 20 (1985), 503–20.

Irvine Loudon, 'The Nature of Provincial Medical Societies in Eighteenth–century England', *Medical History* 27 (1983), 249–68.

R. M. S. McConaghy, 'Medical Ethics in a Changing World', *J. College of General Practitioners* 10 (1965), 3–17.

T. McKeown, 'A Sociological Approach to the History of Medicine', *Medical History* 14 (1970), 342–51.

Angus McLaren, 'Phrenology: Medium and Message', *J. Modern History* 46 (1974), 86–97.

Hilary Marland, 'Early 19th Century Medical Society Activity: The Huddersfield Case', *J. of Regional and Local Studies* 6/2 (1985), 37–48.

W. M. Mathew, 'The Origins and Occupations of Glasgow Students, 1740–1839', *Past and Present* 33 (1966), 74–94.

M. Miller, 'Let the Bow be Unstrung', *Scots Magazine* 105 (1976), 272–6.

J. B. Morrell, 'Reflections on the History of Scottish Science', *History of Science* 12 (1974), 81–94.

——, 'The University of Edinburgh in the Late Eighteenth Century: its Scientific Eminence and Academic Structure', *Isis* 62 (1971), 158–71.

R. H. Nuttall, 'Early Scottish Microscopes', *Medical History* 25 (1981), 199–200.

E. H. L. Oliphant, 'The Royal Faculty of Physicians and Surgeons of Glasgow', *Glasgow Medical Journal* 109 (1928), 152–8.

Katherine Park and Lorraine J. Daston, 'Unnatural Conceptions: The Study of Monsters in Sixteenth and Seventeenth Century France and England', *Past and Present* 92 (1983), 20–53.

Terry Parssinen, 'Popular Science and Society: The Phrenology Movement in Early Victorian Britain', *J. of Social History* (Fall, 1974), 1–20.

M. Jeanne Peterson, 'Gentlemen and Medical Men: The Problem of Professional Recruitment', *Bulletin of the History of Medicine* 58 (1984), 457–73.

Sir Humphry Rolleston, 'Medical Friendships, Clubs and Societies', *Annals of Medical History* 2 (1930), 249–66.

A. Rook, 'Transactions of the Huntingdonshire Medical Society', *Medical History* 4 (1960), 236–52.

Lisa M. Rosner, 'Andrew Duncan MD, FRSE (1744–1828)', (History of Medicine and Science Unit pamphlet, Edinburgh, 1981).

Steven Shapin, 'Property, Patronage, and the Politics of Science: The Founding of the Royal Society of Edinburgh', *Brit. J. of History of Science,* 7 (1974), 1–41.

——, 'The Audience for Science in Eighteenth Century Edinburgh', *History of Science* 12 (1974), 95–121.

——, 'Phrenological Knowledge and the Structure of Early Nineteenth Century Edinburgh', *Annals of Science* 32 (1975), 219–43.

S. E. D. Shortt, 'Physicians, Science and Status: Issues in the Professionalisation of Anglo-American Medicine in the Nineteenth Century', *Medical History* 27 (1983), 51–68.

Stefan Slater, 'The Glasgow Southern Medical Society 100 Years Ago: A Centennial Review', *Bulletin of the Royal College of Physicians and Surgeons Glasgow* 18 (1988), 24–31.

——, 'Further Centennial Reflections on the Glasgow Southern Medical Society', *Bull. Roy. Coll. Phys. Surg. Glas.* 18 (1989), 20–7.

——, '1888–1889, the Year of The Victoria Infirmary: from the Minutes of the Glasgow Southern Medical Society', *Bull. Roy. Coll. Phys. Surg. Glas.* 19 (1990), 22–9.

J. A. Stewart, 'Jubilee of the National Insurance Act', *Pharmaceutical Journal* 189 (1962), 33–5.

P. Swan, 'A Brief Survey and Summary of the Role and Position of Medical Societies in the Early Nineteenth Century Medical Profession', *Jnl of Local Studies* 2/2 (1982), 43–7.

H. P. Tait, 'Notes on the Scottish Branch of the Society of Medical Officers of Health', *Public Health* 90 (1976), 265–70.

T. J. Thomson, 'The Royal Medico-Chirurgical Society of Glasgow – Past and Present', *Scottish Medical Journal* 21 (1976), 168–74.

Charles Edward Underhill, 'Sketch of the History of the Obstetrical Society of Edinburgh', *Edinburgh Medical Journal* 35/2 (1890), 738–47; 831–44.

Ivan Waddington, 'The Development of Medical Ethics – A Sociological Analysis', *Medical History* 27 (1975), 36–51.

THESES AND DISSERTATIONS

Michael Barfoot, 'James Gregory (1753–1821) and Scottish Scientific Metaphysics, 1750–1800', (University of Edinburgh, Ph. D thesis, 1983).

Christopher Lawrence, 'Medicine as Culture: Edinburgh and the Scottish Enlightenment' (University of London, Ph. D thesis, 1984).

Davis D. McElroy, 'The Literary Clubs and Societies of Eighteenth-Century Scotland' (University of Edinburgh, Ph. D. thesis, 1952).

Steven Shapin, 'The Royal Society of Edinburgh: A Study in the Social Context of Hanoverain Science' (University of Pennsylvania, Ph. D. thesis, 1971).

Russell Gordon Smith, 'The Professional Conduct Jurisdiction of the General Medical Council: Its Compliance with Aspects of Substantive and Procedural Justice' (King's College, University of London, Ph. D thesis, 1990).

JOURNALS, NEWSPAPERS AND OTHER CONTEMPORARY PRINTED SOURCES

Aberdeen Journal.
British Medical Journal.
Caledonian Medical Journal.
Chemist and Druggist.
Cook and Wylie's Stirling Directory.
Edinburgh Almanac (and local supplements).
Edinburgh Magazine and Review.
Edinburgh Medical and Surgical Journal.
Edinburgh Medical Journal.
Fife Herald.
Fife Illustrated.
Glasgow Herald.
Glasgow Medical Examiner.
Glasgow Medical Journal.
Glasgow Post Office Directory.
Glasgow University Students' Handbook.
Greenock Trade Directory.

Hansard.
Harvey's Stirling Directory and Almanack.
Inverness Adveriser.
Inverness Journal.
Lancet.
Medical Directory.
Monthly Journal of Medical Science.
Newsletter of the Medical Women's Federation.
Official Year-Book of Scientific and Learned Societies of Great Britain and Ireland.
Pharmaceutical Journal.
Provincial Medical and Surgical Association Journal.
Scots' Magazine.
Stirling Journal and Advertiser.

PRINTED SOCIETY SOURCES CONSULTED

Annals of the Scottish Society of Anaesthetists (Edinburgh, 1989).
Annual Reports of the Forfarshire Medical Association (Dundee, 1898–1927).
Circular for the Medical Practitioners of Fife (Fife Medico-Chirurgical Society) (Cupar, 1828).
Constitution of Glasgow Northern Medical Society (Glasgow, 1903).
Constitution of the Tuberculosis Society of Scotland (Edinburgh, 1921).
First Annual Report of the Glasgow Curative Mesmeric Association (Glasgow, 1862).
First Report of the Medico-Statistical Association (Edinburgh, 1852).
Laws of the Fife Medico-Chirurgical Society (Cupar, 1827).
Laws of the Glasgow Southern Medical Society (11th reprint, Glasgow, 1980).
Laws of the Hunterian Medical Society (Edinburgh, 1840).
Memoirs of the Wernerian Natural History Society, 8 vols (Edinburgh/London 1811–39).
Printed Regulations of the Glasgow and West of Scotland Medical Association (Glasgow, 1875).
Proceedings of the Border Medical Society (Kelso, 1841).
Proceedings of the Edinburgh Obstetrical Society (Edinburgh, 1847).
Proceedings of the Royal Physical Society, vols 1–8 (Edinburgh, 1858–85).
Programme of the Scottish Society for Experimental Medicine Golden Jubilee Meeting, 28th October 1988 (Glasgow, 1988).
Revised Laws of the Edinburgh Medico-Chirurgical Society (Edinburgh, 1869).
Rules of the Clinical Club (Dundee, 1899).
Rules of the Dundee Medical Club (Dundee, 1897).
Table of Fees of the Garioch and Northern Medical Association (Inverurie, 1863).
Transactions of the Botanical Society of Edinburgh vols 1–20 (Edinburgh, 1840–96).
Transactions of the Edinburgh Medico-Chirurgical Society (Edinburgh, 1824 and *passim*).
Transactions of the Edinburgh Obstetrical Society vol. 21 (Edinburgh, 1896).
Transactions of the Forfarshire Medical Association (Dundee, 1924).
Transactions of the Glasgow Pathological and Clinical Society, 11 vols (Glasgow, 1884–1908).
Transactions of the Royal Sanitary Association of Scotland (Glasgow, 1972–82).
Western Infirmary Residents' Club: List of Members 1874 to 1935 (Glasgow, 1935).

Index

Scotland, 21, 123, 198-9
specialisation, medical, 20-2
specialist societies, 8, 9-10, 20-2
Spence, Robert, 152
St Andrews University, 133
St Andrews University Medical Society, 220-1
St Mungo's College Medical Society, 221
Stalker, Alexander Mitchell, 220
state involvement, 97-103
Statistical Society of Glasgow, 199
status
  of medical profession, 14, 85, 86, 103
  of medical societies, 3
Steele, J. C., 165
Stirling, 15
Stirling Medical Association, 199-200
Stirling Medical Society, 200-1
Stirton, James, 221
Strachan, John Mitchell, 80-1, 129, 130
Straton, James, 121
Stratton, Thomas, 149
student medical societies, 14
surgeons, 13, 53-6, 62-3
Syme, James, 42, 141, 171, 201

Tait, John, 212
teratogenesis, 44
Thomson, Emily Charlotte, 94;
Thomson, John (Professor of General
    Pathology, University of Edinburgh,
    c. 1832), 122
Thomson, John (Senior Physician, Royal Sick
    Children's Hospital, Edinburgh,
    c. 1922), 193
Thomson, John Martin (general practitioner,
    Clarkston, c. 1900), 88-90
Town and Country Club, 201
transactions of societies, 26, 30, 35-7, 41-2, 44
transport, 17
Trevelyan, Walter Calverly (Sir), 197
Truck Law Amendment Act, 191
Tuberculosis Society of Scotland, 21, 197
Tuke, John Batty (Sir), 145
Turner, Arthur Logan, 192
Turner, Robert, 125
Turner, William (Sir), 172, 190

University College, Dundee, 134
University of Edinburgh
  American Medical Society, 207
  American Physical Society, 207
  Botanical Society of Edinburgh, 126
  chair of General Pathology, 122
  chair of Midwifery, 40-1
  Chirurgo Medical Society, 209
  Edinburgh Galenian Society, 139
  Edinburgh Medical Missionary Society, 141
  Edinburgh Medical Society, 141
  Edinburgh Pathological Society, 145-6

Edinburgh Phrenological Society, 74, 147
Edinburgh Women's Medical Society, 212
Granton Club, 171
Hibernian Medical Society, 215
Hibernian Physical Society, 215
Hunterian Medical Society, 216
medical faculty, 10
professional elite, 59-61
Scottish Microscopial Society, 190
unqualified practitioners, 55

Vaccination Bill (1880), 153
vaccinations, 54, 158
Victoria Infirmary, 35, 168
voluntary services, 5-6

Walker, Norman, 91, 189, 217
Watson, Ann Mercer, 95
Watt, Ernest, 170
Webster, Alexander, 136
Webster, George, 136
Weir, William, 73, 76, 166
Welsh, John, 186
Werner, Adam Gottlob, 201
Wernerian Natural History Society, 201-2
Western Infirmary Residents' Club, 202
Western Medical Association, 202-3
Western Medical Club, 203-4
widows' funds, 56, 158
Wilson, John, 182
Wise Club, *see* Aberdeen Philosophical Society
Wisemann, Robert, 150
women, 6, 93-7, 107
  Aberdeen University, 206
  Dundee Medical Club, 134
  Edinburgh Obstetrical Society, 144
  Forfarshire Medical Association, 153
  Glasgow Obstetrical and Gynaecological
      Society, 164
  Glasgow Pathological and Clinical Society,
      166
  Glasgow Southern Medical Society, 168
  Glasgow University Medico-Chirurgical
      Society, 213
  Govan Medical Society, 170
  Paisley Medical Society, 182
  Queen Margaret College Medical Society,
      219
  Royal Medico-Chirurgical Society of
      Glasgow, 184
  Scottish Opthalmological Club, 191
  Western Infirmary Residents' Club, 202
Wood, John Robertson, 173
Wood, Winifred, 107, 195
Woodhead, Sims, 145

Yellowlees, John, 45, 149